30 Day Whole Food Challenge

30-Day Whole Food Diet Challenge Recipe Cookbook for Weight Loss

Eat healthy, Lose Weight!

book are for clarifying purposes only and are the owned by the owners themselves, not affiliated with this document.

Table of Contents

Introduction

Nature gifted us her most valuable resources and we should value them as they are, without trying to transform them. For many years, humans lived on the natural nutrients that nature provides us with, but unfortunately, only in the last century food experiments were conducted and implemented to produce crazy amounts of food.

Today, it's increasingly harder to find an ingredient that has naturally grown under the sun. Instead, the food industry giants are continually looking for cheaper ways of producing more and more food for larger profits thus introducing many artificial ingredients into our food.

What does this mean for us?

The sad thing is that, as our schedules become tighter and tighter, most of us are opting for empty-calorie, ready-to-eat foods from these food giants that only require to be popped in the microwave for 3 minutes and voila! Dinner is ready!

Should the ever-increasing cases of lifestyle diseases such as cancer, diabetes, heart diseases, and the like then come as a surprise to us? I will tell you with certainty, NO! If we all stop just for a few seconds and pay attention to what our bodies are saying and respect that, only then will we understand that our bodies need real food to function and heal.

This is where the whole food diet comes in; healthy living is a lifestyle and starting with the whole food diet is the first step to success. When undertaking the whole food diet, you should emphasize on dark green leafy veggies, plant obtained foods and other natural foods that have undergone zero or minimal processing. We are going to look at the whole food diet approved foods, complete with over 100 healthy whole food recipes in this guide.

With the popularity of this diet, what's your excuse for not giving it a shot? Is it the cost, being too busy to make any diet work or the fact that you have a raging sweet tooth? We've all been here so I totally get it. But, with a lot of determination and some planning and keeping things simple, the whole food diet is totally possible.

We are going to look at some delicious recipes made using every day healthy ingredients so don't worry about cost or using too much time cooking. When it comes to all the functions within your body, it all starts with food. So, let's get started!

The Building Blocks of the Whole Food Diet

Food should nourish your entire being!

In a general sense, whole foods are not any different from organic foods. Whole foods refer to any items of consumption that have been subjected to minimal or preferably no processing at all. The 30 Day Whole Food Diet Challenge to Lose Weight principally is based on the ideals of consuming clean, fresh, and healthy and natural foods to make sure of your complete and optimal physiological development.

Where it all started...

Human beings have survived on this planet for over one hundred thousand years and since the beginning of time, have survived on natural, wild growing foods. Our earliest ancestors thrived on wild fruits, veggies, roots and animal flesh and if Paleolithic evidence is anything to go by, they had some of the healthiest bodies.

Where did we take a wrong turn?

It all comes down to economics. In a world where the human population keeps increasing, the demand for food is almost more than the production. As a result, the food industry giants have turned to artificial methods to increase food productivity and reduce the time it takes for plants and animals to grow to maturity.

A very good example is: a normal free range chicken needs months to hatch from an egg and grow into a mature chicken. But, for the last few years, in order to make the chicken bigger and reduce the time of development, a cocktail of antibiotics, hormones and steroids are injected into the chicken eggs to make them disease resistant and so they can be sent to the slaughter house within a month of hatching!

This is just a tip of the iceberg. Many similar trends have been culminating for years which has unfortunately led to the alarming numbers of chronic illnesses including obesity and premature deaths resulting from them.

The question is, why hasn't anyone done anything to stop this madness?

In truth, with the discovery of penicillin and the milestones achieved in medicine and pharmaceuticals, most of us opt for the band aid approach of healing what's on the surface instead of digging deeper to find the root cause of the disease and this is what the whole food diet is all about.

Your body is fully capable of healing itself, all it needs is healthy and natural nutrition to kick-start the healing process.

Why You Should Embark On the 30-Day Whole Food Diet Challenge

- ### Increased fiber intake

The whole food diet pays greater emphasis on fruit and veggies, which are naturally endowed with fiber. Fiber plays an important role in your body by binding to toxins and eliminating them through waste and also improving your digestive function. Some of the foods rich in fiber are almonds, broccoli, brown rice and citrus fruit.

- ### Stay focused all day

With the whole food diet, there no such thing as an afternoon slump because your body is harvesting energy from high quality sources. Natural foods provide you with a slow but steady flow of energy that will keep you alert and focused all day long.

- ### Break the unhealthy chain of food addiction

"I had a terrible day, I need my favorite pick-me-up (ice cream) to cheer me up!" does this sound like you? Well, with the whole food diet, you can say goodbye, once and for all, to your terrible food addictions and obsessions.

The whole food diet rewires your entire system and reminds every single organ in your body that it needs healthy and natural food to provide it with first-grade fuel, not empty calorie foods.

- ### Manage and reverse symptoms of chronic illnesses

The reason why western medicine has failed terribly at curing chronic illnesses is because it only focuses on healing the symptoms and not the disease itself.

A good example is, you are suffering from a food sensitivity, on seeing your GP, you are handed a box of tablets to reduce the discomfort.

The problem with this approach is that it does not address the underlying case of inflammation, which triggered your immune system to respond with inflammation that manifested as a food sensitivity? As with any other health condition, it starts with food!

The whole food diet is comprised of the purest foods that help your body trigger its self-healing ability to combat even the most serious of health conditions.

- **Having a problem with your reproductive function?**

The typical Western diet is laden with artificial ingredients that are doused with chemicals, some of which mimic the hormone estrogen. For women, the body is fooled into thinking that there is enough estrogen and so it withholds itself from releasing estrogen therein affecting your fertility.

Ever seen men with boobs (moobs), this is because the estrogen-mimicking chemicals cause the men to have a higher level of 'estrogen' than they should have and as a result have lower testosterone levels.

The whole food diet reboots your entire system thus restoring normalcy in your endocrine function.

- **`Discover the fountain of youth**

You will be surprised at how clear and radiant your skin looks after 30 days of no junk; and not just your skin but also hair and nails. Your skin is a mirror of how healthy you are. By cutting out all processed foods, your skin will be the perfect picture of health.

- **No more sleepless nights**

Perhaps the greatest benefit of the whole food diet is that it regulates your hormone patterns meaning your body will stay awake when it should and completely shut down when it's supposed to. Additionally, your body heals and repairs all damaged tissues at night. With a healthy and nutritious diet, you can expect a lot of healing and repairing.

We can't possibly exhaust all the benefits of the whole food diet. We leave the rest up to you, give it an honest try and you will feel reborn!

The 30-Day Whole Food Diet Challenge Meal Plan

DAY	BREAKFAST	AM SNACK	LUNCH	PM SNACK	DINNER	BEDTIME
DAY 1	1 Serving Rhubarb-Oatmeal Porridge	Sesame Crackers 1 glass (250ml) coconut water	1 Serving Superfood Sushi	1 glass (250ml) Lemon Juice	1 Serving Liver and Onions	1 serving Pickled Veggies
DAY 2	1 Serving Citrus Granola Parfait	1 serving Squash Fries	1 Serving The Ultimate Kale Salad	1 serving Stuffed Celery Bites	1 Serving Fried Salmon Fillets	1 glass (250ml) Basil, Ginger, and Lemon Iced Tea

DAY 3	1 Serving Blueberry Oatmeal Waffles 1 glass (250ml) Apple Lemonade	A handful of mixed berries (blueberries ,raspberries, blackberries ,strawberries)	1 bowl Butternut Squash Soup	1 Serving Carrot French Fries	1 Serving Lemongrass and Chilli Beef	1 serving Healthy Spiced Nuts
DAY 4	1 Serving Toast w/ Refried Beans & Avocado	1 apple sprinkled with cinnamon	1 Serving Kale Avocado Salad with Orange	1 serving Pesto-Stuffed Mushrooms	1 Serving Vegetarian Curry	1 Glass Spiced Tea
DAY 5	6 Healthy Banana Cookies 1 glass Lemon Juice	1 Serving Squash Fries	1 Serving Spinach and Beet Salad	1 glass (250ml) Apple Lemonade	1 Serving Orange-Cranberry Crusted Salmon	1 serving Guacamole w/ Vegetables

DAY 6	1 Cup Oatmeal-Strawberry Breakfast Smoothie	1 Serving Vegan Beet Burgers	1 Serving Thai Beef Wraps	Handful Brazil nuts 1 apple sprinkled with cinnamon	1 Serving Chicken Bruschetta	1 Serving Healthy Spiced Nuts
DAY 7	1 Bowl Tapioca Coconut Porridge	Sesame Crackers 1 glass (250ml) coconut water	1 Serving Salmon w/ Chanterelle Mushrooms	1 glass (250ml) Grapefruit Cranberry Sparkler	1 Serving Shrimp Salad w/ Grapefruit and Avocado	1 serving Veggie Snack
DAY 8	1 Serving Grain-Free Muesli	1 glass (250ml) Raspberry Lemonade	1 Serving Hamburger Veggie Casserole	1 Serving Lime Coconut Fizz Cooler	1 Serving Salmon Salad	1 glass (250ml) Catechin-Rich Ice Tea
DAY 9	1 Cup Orange Flax Smoothie	1 Serving Candied Macadamia Nuts	1 Serving Red Snapper in Sauce	1 glass (250ml) Hydration JuiceSmoothie	1 Serving 1 Serving Beetroot and Carrot Burgers	1 glass Orange Juice

DAY 10	4 Chewy Baked Granola Bars 1 glass (250ml) orange juice	1 Serving Squash w/ Cherries	1 Serving Chickpea Salad	1 Serving Sesame Crackers	1 Serving Lemongrass and Chilli Beef	1glass (250ml) Apple Lemonade
DAY 11	1 Serving Citrus Granola Parfait	1 serving Stuffed Mushrooms	1 Serving Coconut Chicken w/ Mustard-Honey Sauce	1 Serving Healthy Spiced Nuts	1 Serving Warm Lemon Chicken	1 glass orange juice
DAY 12	1 Serving Nutty Cinnamon Quinoa	1 Serving Vegan Beet Burgers	1 Serving Mustard Crusted Salmon with Arugula and Spinach Salad	1 glass (250ml) Raspberry Lemonade	1 Serving Warm Lemon Chicken	1 Serving Kale Chips

DAY 13	1 Serving Superfood Detox Pancakes 1 glass (250ml) Apple Lemonade	1 Serving Veggie Snack	1 Serving Green Super Detox Salad	1 Serving Candied Macadamia Nuts	1 Serving Chicken w/Peppers	Sesame Crackers 1 glass (250ml) coconut water
DAY 14	1 Serving Oat Muesli with Raspberries and Apples	1 glass Lemon Juice	1 Bowl Broccoli Detox Soup	1 glass Basil, Ginger and Lemon Iced Tea	1 Serving Coconut Chicken	1Serving Healthy Spiced Nuts
DAY 15	1 Serving Healthy Multigrain Cereal	1 Serving Cacao Smoothie w/ Macadamias	1 Serving Spinach Strawberry Salad	1 Serving Veggie Snack	1 Serving Turkey & Quinoa Salad	1 glass (250ml) Raspberry Lemonade

DAY 16	1 Bowl Buckwheat-Pumpkin Power Porridge	1 glass (250ml) Apple Lemonade	1 Serving Chickpea Salad w/ Zucchini & Avocado Mayo	1 Serving Roasted Asparagus	1 Serving Warm Lemon Chicken	1 Serving Kale Chips
DAY 17	1 Serving Sunflower Oat Breakfast Bars 1 glass (250ml) Orange Juice	1 Serving Carrot French Fries	1 Bowl Cleansing Detox Soup	1 Piece Spinach Cake	1 Serving Cauliflower Pizza	1 glass (250ml) Strawberry Lemonade
DAY 18	1 Serving Poached Eggs over Mushrooms and Spinach	Squash Fries	1 Serving Citrus and Spinach Salad	1 Serving Stuffed Celery Bites	1 Serving Chicken Bruschetta	1 Glass Apple Lemonade
DAY 19	1 Cup Healthy Breakfast Granola	1 glass strawberry lemonade	1 Bowl Chilled Green Goddess Soup	1 Serving Kale Chips	1 Serving Fried Salmon Fillets	1 Cup Easy Guacamole + Carrot sticks

DAY 20	1 Serving Buckwheat and Oat Muesli with Grapes and Pears	1 glass (250ml) Orange Juice	1 Serving Avocado Grapefruit Edamame Salad	1 Serving Carrot French Fries	1 Serving Salmon Salad	1 Serving Baked Cinnamon Apple Chips
DAY 21	1 Serving Grain-Free Muesli	1 Serving Vinegar & Salt Kale Chips	1 Serving The Ultimate Kale Salad	Sesame Crackers 1 glass (250ml) coconut water	1 Serving Warm Lemon Chicken	1 glass lemon juice
DAY 22	1 Cup Oatmeal-Strawberry Breakfast Smoothie	1 cup Easy Guacamole + Celery sticks	1 Serving Roasted Power Bowl w/ Lemon Tahini Dressing	1 Serving Lemon Juice	1 Serving Beetroot and Carrot Burgers	1 Piece Spinach Cake
DAY 23	1 Serving Superfood Granola	1 Serving Cacao Smoothie w/ Macadamias	1 Serving Kale Avocado Salad with Orange	1 glass Orange juice	1 Serving Coconut Chicken	Toasted cashew nuts

DAY 24	1 Serving Beet Quinoa w/ Orange	1 Serving Candied Macadamia Nuts	1 Bowl Carrot and Goji Berry Soup	1 Piece Spinach Cake	1 Serving Warm Lemon Chicken	1 glass lemon juice
DAY 25	1 Serving Oat Muesli with Raspberries and Apples	Toasted pumpkin seeds	1 Serving Salad For Glowing Skin + Detox Dressing	1 Serving Carrot French Fries	1 Serving Chicken w/Peppers	1 glass orange juice
DAY 26	1 Cup Goji Berry, Raspberry, Apple, and Kale Smoothie	1 Serving Vinegar & Salt Kale Chips	1 Bowl Healthy Detox Soup	1 Serving Roasted Balsamic Beets	1 Serving Liver and Onions	1 glass (250ml) Strawberry Lemonade
DAY 27	1 Bowl Buckwheat Porridge	1 Piece Spinach Cake	1 Serving Lemony Asparagus & Tomato Salad	1 glass (250ml) Raspberry Lemonade	1 Serving Shrimp Salad w/ Grapefruit and Avocado	1 Serving Roasted Sweet Potato Chips

DAY 28	1 Serving Avocado Superfood Tapenade & Egg Toast 1 glass (250ml) Lemon Juice	Sesame Crackers 1 glass (250ml) coconut water	1 Bowl Healthy Detox Soup	1 Serving Baked Cinnamon Apple Chips	1 Serving Salmon Salad	1 apple sprinkled with cinnamon
DAY 29	1 Serving Avocado Toast w/ Poached Egg 1 glass (250ml) orange juice	1 Serving Veggie Snack	1 Serving Cauliflower Couscous Salad	1 glass Matcha Pineapple Mango Smoothie	1 Serving Lemongrass and Chilli Beef	1 glass raspberry Lemonade
DAY 30	1 Cup Detox Breakfast Smoothie	1 glass Apple Lemonade	1 Serving Swiss Chard Wrap	1 glass Liver Detox Juice	1 Serving Vegetarian Curry	Sesame Crackers 1 glass (250ml) coconut water

Whole Food Diet Recipes

Whole Food Breakfast Recipes

Blueberry Oatmeal Waffles

Yield: 6 (8-inch) Waffles

Total Time: 20 Minutes

Prep Time: 15 Minutes

Cook Time: 5 Minutes

Ingredients

- 1 1/2 cups frozen blueberries
- 1 1/2 cups almond milk
- 1/3 cup applesauce
- 1 cup quick cooking oats
- 1 cup whole-wheat flour
- 2 tbsp. canola oil
- 1/4 tsp. ground allspice
- 2 tbsp. raw honey
- 1/2 tsp. sea salt
- 1 tsp. pure vanilla extract
- 1 tbsp. baking powder

Directions

In a mixing bowl, sift together flour, allspice, baking powder, and sat; stir in oats and make a well in the center. Add oil, honey, milk, applesauce, and vanilla in the well and stir until well combined. Set aside the batter to rest for at least 5 minutes or until slightly thickened; fold in the blueberries.

Cook the waffles in the waffle iron, following manufacturer's instructions.

Toast w/ Refried Beans & Avocado

Yield: 2 Servings

Total Time: 15 Minutes

Prep Time: 5 Minutes

Cook Time: 10 Minutes

Ingredients

- 2 slices bread
- 1 cup homemade refried beans
- 1 avocado, thinly sliced
- Slivered white onion
- Sea salt

Directions

Toast the bread to your liking. Top with the refried beans and avocado slices; scatter with silvered onions and sprinkle with salt to serve.

Nutty Cinnamon Quinoa

Yield: 4 Servings

Total Time: 25 Minutes

Prep Time: 10 Minutes

Cook time: 15 Minutes

Ingredients

- 1 cup quinoa
- 1 cup almond milk
- 1/3 cup chopped toasted pecans
- 1/2 tsp. ground cinnamon
- 2 cups fresh blackberries
- 1 cup water
- 4 tsp. raw honey

Directions

In a medium saucepan, combine milk, quinoa, and water; bring to a rolling boil over high heat. Lower heat to medium low and simmer, covered, for about 15 minutes or until almost all liquid is absorbed. Remove from heat and stir in cinnamon and strawberries.

Divide the quinoa among four servings bowl and top each with pecans; drizzle with a teaspoon of honey and serve.

Citrus Granola Parfait

Yield: 4 Servings

Total Time: 45 Minutes

Prep Time: 10 Minutes

Cook time: 30 Minutes

Ingredients:

- 16 ounces vanilla soy yogurt
- 1/8 cup dried cranberries
- 1/8 cup dried apricots, chopped
- 1/8 cup flax seed
- 1/8 cup unsweetened dried coconut
- 1/8 cup almonds, chopped
- 1/8 cup raw walnuts, chopped
- 1/8 cup sunflower seeds
- 1/8 cup pumpkin seeds
- 1 cup rolled oats
- 1 1/2 tbsp. grape seed oil
- 2 tbsp. each of lemon, orange, and lime juice
- 1 tbsp. each of lemon, orange, and lime zest
- 1/2 tsp. vanilla extract
- 1 1/2 tbsp. raw honey

Directions

Preheat your oven to 300°F.

In a large bowl, combine all ingredients except yogurt; stir until well combined. Spread the mixture onto a cookie sheet and bake for about 15 minutes. Stir and continue baking for 15 minutes more.

Remove the granola from oven and let cool to room temperature.

Alternate the scoops of granola with the scoops of soy yogurt until the serving bowl is full. Enjoy!

Chewy Baked Granola Bars

Yield: 10-12 Bars

Total Time: 35 Minutes

Prep Time: 10 Minutes

Cook Time: 25 Minutes

Ingredients:

- 3/4 cup oatmeal
- 1/4 cup dried cranberries, chopped
- 1/4 cup raw pumpkin seeds
- 1/4 cup raw sunflower seeds
- 1/2 cup chia seeds
- 3/4 cup pitted dates
- 1 tsp. pure vanilla extract
- 1 tsp. cinnamon
- 1 cup water
- 1/4 tsp. sea salt

Directions:

Preheat your oven to 325°F. Line a 9-inch baking pan with 2 parchment papers.

Add oatmeal to a large bowl.

Add water and dates to the blender and let soak for at least 30 minutes; blend until smooth.

Add all the ingredients to the bowl with oatmeal and mix well.

Scoop the oat mixture into the prepared pan and spread out with a spatula; bake for about 25 minutes or until firm when touched. Remove from oven and cool for about 5 minutes before transferring to a cooling rack; let cool completely and the slice.

Rhubarb-Oatmeal Porridge

Yield: 2 Servings

Total Time: 25 Minutes

Prep Time: 20 Minutes

Cook Time: 5 Minutes

Ingredients

- 1 cup 1/2-inch pieces frozen rhubarb
- 1 1/2 cups almond milk
- 2 tbsp. chopped toasted pecans
- 1 cup rolled oats
- 1/2 cup orange juice
- 1/2 tsp. ground cinnamon
- Pinch of salt
- 2 tbsp. raw honey

Directions

In a medium saucepan, combine rhubarb, oats, juice, milk, cinnamon, and salt; bring to a gentle boil over medium heat; lower heat to medium-low and cook, stirring constantly, 5 minutes or until rhubarb and oats until tender.

Remove the pan from heat and let stand covered, for at least 5 minutes; stir in honey and top with nuts to serve.

Orange Flax Smoothie

Yield: 3 Cups

Total Time: 5 Minutes

Prep Time: 5 Minutes

Cook Time: N/A

Ingredients

- 1 cup orange juice
- 1 cup carrot juice
- 2 cups frozen peach slices
- 1 tbsp. chopped fresh ginger
- 2 tbsp. ground flaxseed

Directions

In a blender, combine orange juice, carrot juice, peaches, ginger, and flaxseed; blend until very smooth. Serve immediately.

Tapioca Coconut Porridge

Yield: 4 Servings

Total Time: 50 Minutes

Prep Time: 5 Minutes

Cook Time: 45 Minutes

Ingredients:

- 1/4 cup tapioca

- 2 cups coconut milk

- 2 tbsp. raw honey

- 1 1/2 tsp. lemon juice

- 1/2 cup toasted coconut flakes

Directions

Soak tapioca I 2 cups of water into a heavy-bottomed saucepan for about 30 minutes; add raw honey and coconut milk and bring to a gentle boil over medium heat, stirring. Lower heat and simmer for about 15 minutes or until tapioca is cooked through and translucent.

Remove from heat and stir in lemon juice; garnish with coconut flakes to serve.

Healthy Banana Cookies

Yield: 4 Servings

Total Time: 30 Minutes

Prep Time: 10 Minutes

Cook time: 20 Minutes

Ingredients

- 1/3 cup extra virgin olive oil
- 1 cup pitted and chopped dates
- 2 cups rolled oats
- 3 ripe bananas
- 1 tsp. vanilla extract

Directions

Preheat oven to 175°C (350°F).

Mash the bananas in a large bowl until very smooth. Stir in vanilla, oil, dates and oats until well combined. Let the mixture sit for at least 15 minutes.

Drop the mixture, by spoonfuls, onto a coated cookie sheet and bake until lightly brown, for about 20 minutes.

Grain-Free Muesli

Yield: 4 Servings

Total Time: 5 Minutes

Prep Time: 5 Minutes

Cook Time: N/A

Ingredients

- ½ cup unsweetened coconut flakes
- ½ cup mixed dried fruit (apple, cranberry, and apricot)
- 3 cups mixed seeds (pumpkin, sunflower, chia, and hemp)
- ½ cup non-dairy milk (coconut, almond, cashew, or hemp)
- 1 banana, sliced
- ½ cup fresh berries (raspberries, blueberries, or strawberries)

Directions

Combine the dry ingredients in a large bowl; mix thoroughly. Stir in milk until well combined. Top your cereal with sliced banana and fresh berries. Enjoy!

Buckwheat and Oat Muesli with Grapes and Pears

Yield: 4 Servings

Total Time: 20 Minutes

Prep Time: 10 Minutes

Cook time: 10 Minutes

Ingredients

- 1/2 cup puffed buckwheat
- 1 1/2 cups rolled oats
- 1 cup halved red grapes
- 1 cup diced organic pears
- 1/2 cup chopped dried apples
- 1 tbsp. honey
- 2 tsp. ground cinnamon
- Rice milk

Directions

Preheat your oven to 325°F.

Evenly spread the oats onto a baking tray and toast in the oven, stirring occasionally, for about 10 minutes.

Remove the oats from oven and set aside to cool.

When cool, transfer the oats to a glass bowl or a ceramic bowl and add water. Soak in the refrigerator for at least 8 hours or overnight.

Stir in brown honey, cinnamon, dried apples and puffed buckwheat until the sugar is completely dissolved.

Divide the mixture among the serving bowl and top with grapes and pears. Serve with rice milk for a healthy, satisfying breakfast.

Quinoa Breakfast Cereal with Almonds and Berries

Yield: 4 Servings

Total Time: 28 Minutes

Prep Time: 10 Minutes

Cook time: 18 Minutes

Ingredients:

- 1 cup rinsed and dried quinoa

- 1 3/4 cup coconut milk

- 2 tsp. raw honey

- A pinch of salt

- 1 cup rinsed and halved organic berries

- 1/2 cup roughly chopped raw almonds

Directions

Bring coconut milk to a gentle boil in a large pot; stir in quinoa.

Reduce heat to low and simmer until quinoa is plump, for about 18 minutes.

Stir in the honey and serve with chopped almonds and berries and more coconut milk, if desired.

Healthy Breakfast Granola

Yield: 2 Cups

Total Time: 38 Minutes

Prep Time: 15 Minutes

Cook time: 23 Minutes

Ingredients

- 1/8 cup flax meal
- 1 1/4 cups rolled oats
- 2 tsp. canola oil
- 1 tsp. cinnamon
- 4 tbsp. honey
- 1/4 cup apple juice
- Pinch of salt

Directions

Preheat your oven to 325°F.

Coat a baking sheet with canola oil and set aside.

In a bowl, combine together flax meal, oats, cinnamon and salt.

In a separate bowl, combine apple juice and honey.

Stir the wet ingredients into the dry ingredients until well blended and moist.

Evenly spread the mixture into the prepared baking sheet; bake for about 15 minutes.

Remove the baking sheet from the oven and stir to break large chunks into smaller chunks. Continue baking for 8 more minutes or until crisp. Cool and break up the remaining chunks into small pieces. Store granola in airtight container.

Goji Berry, Raspberry, Apple, and Kale Smoothie

Yield: 3 Servings

Total Time: 5 Minutes

Prep Time: 5 Minutes

Cook time: N/A

Ingredients

- 1/3 cup goji berries
- 1 cup raspberries
- 1 apple, chopped
- 2 handfuls fresh kale
- 1 frozen banana
- 1 cup almond milk
- 6 ice cubes

Directions

Combine all ingredients in a blender and blend until very smooth. Enjoy!

Oat Muesli with Raspberries and Apples

Yield: 4 Servings

Total Time: 20 Minutes

Prep Time: 10 Minutes

Cook time: 10 Minutes

Ingredients

- 1/2 cup popped rice
- 1 1/2 cups rolled oats
- 1 cup raspberries
- 1 cup organic apples, diced
- 2 tsp. ground cinnamon
- 2 tbsp. honey
- Rice milk

Directions

Preheat your oven to 325°F.

In a bowl, mix together oats, cinnamon and honey; spread the mixture onto a baking tray; toast in the oven, stirring occasionally, for about 10 minutes.

Remove the oat mixture from the oven and let stand to cool.

Transfer to a bowl and stir in popped rice.

Divide the mixture among serving bowls and top with raspberries and apples. Serve with rice milk.

Poached Eggs over Mushrooms and Spinach

Yield: 3 Servings

Total Time: 22 Minutes

Prep Time: 10 Minutes

Cook time: 12 Minutes

Ingredients:

- 4 free-range eggs
- 10 oz. spinach, thawed
- 3 medium cloves garlic
- 1 medium tomato, chopped
- 2 cups chopped crimini mushrooms
- ½ medium onion
- 1 tbsp. vegetable or broth
- 1 tsp. light vinegar
- Salt
- Pepper

Directions:

Chop garlic and onion; let sit for at least 5 minutes.

In the meantime, bring water to a rolling boil in a skillet. Add a teaspoon of vinegar.

Heat broth in a separate skillet. Stir in mushrooms and onion and cook for about 3 minutes over medium heat. Stir in spinach, garlic, tomato, pepper and salt and cook for 3 more minutes.

Add the egg in the boiling water and poach for at least 5 minutes. Remove the egg from the boiling water and place over the spinach mixture.

Healthy Multigrain Cereal

Yield: 2 Servings

Total Time: 15 Minutes

Prep Time: 10 Minutes

Cook time: 5 Minutes

Ingredients

- 2 tbsp. old-fashioned oats

- 2 tbsp. bulgur

- 2 tbsp. barley (quick-cooking)

- 1 tbsp. chopped walnuts

- 1 pinch ground cinnamon

- 2 tbsp. raisins

- ½ cup water

Directions

Combine oats, bulgur, barley and water in a microwave-safe bowl. Microwave on high for about 2 minutes. Stir in cinnamon and raisins and continue heating for 3 more minutes.

Stir and top with walnuts to serve.

Sunflower Oat Breakfast Bars

Yield: 4 Servings

Total Time: 25 Minutes

Prep Time: 10 Minutes

Cook time: 15 Minutes

Ingredients

- 4 cups gluten-free rolled oats
- 2 tbsp. raw honey
- 1 cup sunflower seed oil
- 1/2 cup dried blueberries
- 1 cup diced dried banana
- 1 tsp. kosher salt
- 2 tsp. ground cinnamon
- 1 cup sunflower seeds (raw)

Directions

In a bowl, combine all the dry ingredients. Stir in honey and sunflower seed oil. Transfer the mixture to a square pan and press to fit well. Refrigerate until firm. Remove from pan and cut into bars.

Superfood Detox Pancakes

Yield: 1 Serving

Total Time: 15-17 Minutes

Prep Time: 5 Minutes

Cook Time: 10-12 Minutes

Ingredients

- 1/3 cup rolled oats
- 1/2 tsp. cinnamon
- 1/2 tsp. baking powder
- 2 tbsp. ground flax
- 1/2 medium ripe banana
- 3 large egg whites
- 2 cups spinach
- 1/2 tsp. vanilla extract

Directions

Set a nonstick skillet over medium heat; coat with olive oil cooking spray.

In a food processor or blender, blend the oats into fine flour; transfer to a bowl and stir in the remaining dry ingredients.

In a blender, combine banana, egg whites, spinach, and vanilla and blend until very smooth.

Add the banana mixture into the dry ingredients and stir to form batter.

Spoon batter onto the heated skillet, forming four pancakes. Cook for about 6 minutes per side or until browned.

Transfer the pancakes to a plate and top with fresh fruit and nuts.

Buckwheat-Pumpkin Power Porridge

Yield: 2 Servings

Total Time: 15 Minutes

Prep Time: 5 Minutes

Cook Time: 10 Minutes

Ingredients

- 1 cup unsweetened almond milk
- 1/2 cup buckwheat groats, soaked
- 1 ripe banana, sliced
- 1 tsp. vanilla
- 1 tsp. cinnamon + more for topping
- 1/2 cup canned pumpkin
- 1/2 tsp. pumpkin pie spice
- Dried fruit, chia seeds, and nuts for topping

Directions

Place buckwheat groats in a pot and add enough almond milk to cover the groats. Stir in banana slices and cook over medium heat for about 7 minutes or until all the milk has been absorbed.

Stir in vanilla, cinnamon, pumpkin, and pumpkin spice; continue cooking to your desired texture.

Divide the porridge between two serving bowls and sprinkle with toppings. Enjoy!

Superfood Granola

Yield: 5 Cups (6 Servings)

Total Time: 3 Hours 20 Minutes + Soaking Time

Prep Time: 20 Minutes

Cook Time: 3 Hours

Ingredients:

- 1 1/2 cups soaked almonds and walnuts (or any of your favorites)
- 1 cup soaked sunflower seeds or a mix with pumpkin
- 2 cup soaked whole buckwheat (min 4hrs) preferably sprouted for 1-2 days
- 3 grated apple, (strain some of the juice from the grated apple)
- 1/2 cup pureed dates soaked for about 15 minutes
- 1/4 cup dried prunes
- 1/2 cup goji berries soaked for min minutes
- 1/2 cup dry coconut flakes
- 1 tsp. vanilla
- 3 tsp. cinnamon
- 1/3 tsp. salt
- 1 tsp. cacao nibs
- 1 tbsp. of hulled Hemp seeds

Instructions

Soak buckwheat for a minimum of 4 hours and rinse thoroughly.

Soak all the nuts and seeds a minimum 4 hours and rinse.

Soak dates in water enough to cover for a minimum of 15 minutes or until soft.

Soak the Goji berries in sufficient water to cover.

Chop or lightly put through your food processor the nuts and seeds. Maybe leave some whole or until your desired consistency.

Once all ingredients are soaked, rinse and add all together in a large bowl and mix well, use your hands for easiest method.

Take the mixture and spread evenly over a baking trays and cook for 2-3 hours at 200°F/95°C, or until dry. You may use a higher temperature for a quicker cook. To make this recipe raw, you may use a dehydrator at 105° F/55°C for 12-15 hours (turning over when the top is totally dry).

Once completely dry you can store in airtight container for a couple of weeks.

Serve with a nut or seed milk or eat as a snack dry.

Avocado Toast w/ Poached Egg

Yield: 1 Serving

Total Time: 9 Minutes

Prep Time: 5 Minutes

Cook Time: 4 Minutes

Ingredients:

- 1 avocado
- 1 egg
- Gluten-free toast of your choice
- 1/4 of red chili or chili flakes
- Lemon (optional)
- Sea salt and black pepper, to taste

Instructions

Slice your avocado and spread over your toast. Squeeze a little lemon over the avocado, top with poached egg. Sprinkle a little chile on top and serve.

Beet Quinoa w/ Orange

Yield: 2 Servings

Total Time: 30 Minutes

Prep Time: 10 Minutes

Cook time: 20 Minutes

Ingredients

- ½ red onion thinly sliced
- 1 tbsp. apple cider vinegar
- 2-3 beets
- 1 cup quinoa
- 1 stalk celery, thinly sliced
- 1 tsp. grated ginger
- Extra virgin olive oil
- Juice of 1 lemon
- 1 small orange, thinly sliced
- ½ tsp. sea salt
- ½ tsp. freshly ground black pepper

Directions

Combine sliced onion and apple cider vinegar in a bowl; let soak for at least 10 minutes.

In the meantime, bring a pot of water to a gentle boil over medium heat. Rinse the beets and add to the boiling water; boil for about 10 minutes or until tender cooked, but not mushy.

Transfer the beets to a plate and reserve the cooking liquid; peel the cooked beets and chop thinly.

Follow package instructions to cook quinoa using the reserved beet liquid. Season with salt while cooking. When cooked, remove the quinoa from heat and set aside to cool.

In a large serving bowl, mix beets, quinoa, ginger and celery. Remove onion from the vinegar and stir into the bowl with the quinoa mixture.

Drizzle with extra virgin olive oil and lemon juice. Add orange slices and toss to mix well.

Season with salt and pepper to serve.

Buckwheat Porridge

Yield: 2 Servings

Total Time: 25 Minutes

Prep Time: 20 Minutes

Cook time: 5 Minutes

Ingredients

- ½ cup roasted buckwheat
- pinch cinnamon
- 1 cup non-dairy milk (almond, coconut, soy, seed)
- 2 tbsp. chia seed
- 1 tsp. vanilla
- small handful large raisins
- 1 red apple, grated
- Dried goji and fresh blueberries to serve
- Honey, optional

Directions

In a large bowl, mix buckwheat, cinnamon, milk, chia, vanilla, and raisins; stir and refrigerate for at least 8 hours or overnight. Stir in grated apple and cook over medium-low heat for about 5 minutes or until creamy and thick. Stir in honey, if using, and add more milk if necessary.

Serve porridge in bowls topped with goji and blueberries.

Detox Breakfast Smoothie

Yield: 4 Servings

Total Time: 10 Minutes

Prep Time: 10 Minutes

Cook time: N/A

Ingredients:

- 2 cups frozen blueberries
- 1 tsp. spirulina powder
- 1 scoop protein powder
- Juice of 1 lemon
- 1 cup organic coconut milk

Topping:

- 1 tbsp. goji berries
- 2 tbsp. milled flax seed
- 1 tbsp. chia seed

Directions:

Combine smoothie ingredients in a blender and blend until very smooth. Serve the smoothie in a bowl topped with your favorite topping and enjoy!

Apple & Cinnamon Porridge

Yield: 4 Servings

Total Time: 22 Minutes

Prep Time: 15 Minutes

Cook time: 7 Minutes

Ingredients

- 1 apple, peeled, cored and chopped
- 1 tsp. raw honey
- 200g porridge oats or oatmeal
- 400ml soy milk
- 800ml water
- 1 tsp. ground cinnamon
- Pinch of salt
- Raisins or currants, to serve

Directions

Combine apple, honey and a splash of water in a pan over medium heat; cook for about 10 minutes or until apple is tender cooked. Transfer to a bowl along with the cooking liquid and set aside.

Add oats, soymilk, and cinnamon to the pan and bring to a gentle boil, stirring continuously.

Reduce the heat to medium low and simmer for about 7 minutes or until it reaches your desired consistency.

Cover with a lid and allow to rest for five minutes, then stir in the apple puree.

Serve topped with sugar, extra milk and a few currants or raisins.

Avocado Superfood Tapenade & Egg Toast

Yield: 2 Servings

Total Time: 5 Minutes

Prep Time: 5 Minutes

Cook Time: N/A

Ingredients

- Gluten-free toasts
- 2 tsp. tahini
- 1 ripe avocado, peeled and cut into slices
- 2 free-range eggs, poached
- 2 tsp. chia seeds
- 2 tsp. pumpkin seeds
- 2 tbsp. superfood tapenade

For the tapenade

- 2 tsp. extra virgin olive oil
- 1 tbsp. lemon juice
- 1 garlic clove
- ½ tsp. spirulina
- 1 tsp. pumpkin seeds
- ½ cup green pitted olives
- 1 cup fresh kale leaves
- A pinch sea salt

Directions

Drizzle tahini sauce over the toasts and add avocado slices; top with poached egg.

In a blender, pulse the tapenade ingredients until very smooth and store in an airtight container; add two tablespoons of the tapenade over the toast and garnish with chia and pumpkin seeds. Serve right away.

Whole Food Lunch Recipes

Swiss Chard Wrap

Total Time: 20 Minutes

Yield: 4 Servings

Total Time: 20 Minutes

Prep Time: 20 Minutes

Cook Time: 0 Minutes

Ingredients

- 4 large Swiss chard leaves
- 1 red bell pepper
- 1 avocado
- ¼ -1/3 cups (2-3 ounces) alfalfa sprouts
- 1 carrot
- 1 cucumber
- ½ lime
- 1/4 cup raw pecans
- 1 tbsp. tamari (gluten-free soy sauce)
- 1 tsp. cumin
- ½ tsp. minced garlic
- ½ tsp. grated ginger
- 1 tsp. extra virgin olive oil
- Handful of alfalfa sprouts

Directions

To prepare Swiss chard, wash leaves, cut off stiff white stem at the bottom and slice thinly to be added to each wrap. Or Juiced! Dry the leaves off with paper towels and using a knife thinly slice down the central root (to make it easier to bend the leaves for wrapping).

Thinly slice all vegetables.

In a food processor, combine pecans, tamari, cumin, garlic, ginger and olive oil. Pulse until combined.

Place a collard leaf in front of you and layer nut mix, red pepper slices, avocado slices, cucumber, carrot and a drizzle of lime juice and alfalfa sprouts. Then wrap up the sides. I

sometimes use a toothpick to keep the wrap together if it decides to unwrap.

Avocado Grapefruit Edamame Salad

Yield: 3 Servings

Total Time: 10 Minutes

Prep Time: 10 Minutes

Cook time: N/A

For the Salad

- 1 small (or half of a large) ripe avocado, peeled and sliced
- 2 celery stalks, sliced
- 1 cup shelled edamame
- 1 blood orange, segmented
- 1 grapefruit, segmented
- 2 cups leafy greens

For the Dressing

- 1/4 cup (2 unces) plus 1 tablespoon extra virgin olive oil
- 2 tbsp. apple cider vinegar
- 1 tbsp. gluten-free mustard
- 1 tbsp. raw honey
- 3 tbsp. diced shallots
- Sea salt and cracked black pepper, to taste

Directions

Combine all salad ingredients in a medium bowl.

Combine extra virgin olive oil, vinegar, mustard, raw honey, shallots, salt and pepper in a jar with a tight fitting lid; seal and shake until well blended.

Pour enough dressing over the salad and season with salt and pepper. Serve right away!

Spinach Strawberry Salad

Yields: 4 Servings

Total Time: 15 Minutes

Prep Time: 15 Minutes

Cook Time: N/A

Ingredients

- 1 quart hulled and sliced strawberries
- 10 ounces fresh spinach – chopped
- 1 tbsp. minced onion
- 1 tbsp. poppy seeds
- 2 tbsp. sesame seeds
- 1/4 tsp. Worcestershire sauce
- 1/4 tsp. paprika
- 1/4 cup distilled white vinegar
- 1/2 cup extra virgin olive oil
- 1 tbsp. raw honey
- 1/4 cup silvered almonds, blanched

Directions

In a bowl, whisk together extra virgin olive oil, poppy seeds, honey, sesame seeds, onion, Worcestershire sauce, paprika and vinegar; cover and chill for at least 1 hour.

In a separate bowl, combine almonds, strawberries and spinach; pour the chilled dressing over the salad and toss until well coated; chill for about 10 minutes before serving.

Chickpea Salad

Yields: 4 Servings

Total Time: 5 Minutes

Prep Time: 5 Minutes

Cook Time: N/A

Ingredients

- 1 tbsp. lemon juice
- 1 tbsp. mashed avocado
- ½ onion, diced
- 1 stalk celery, diced
- 1 15.5-oz can chickpeas
- 1 tsp. dried dill
- Salt
- Pepper

Directions

Sauté onion in a pan set over medium heat until translucent.

Mash chickpeas in a small bowl until smooth. Add sautéed onion, celery, mashed avocado, lemon juice and dill; stir until well combined.

Season with ground pepper and salt to taste.

Spinach and Beet Salad

Yields: 4 Servings

Total Time: 17 Minutes

Prep Time: 10 Minutes

Cook Time: 7 Minutes

Ingredients

- 1 tbsp. extra-virgin olive oil
- 2 cups beet wedges, steamed
- 8 cups baby spinach
- 2 tbsp. sliced Kalamata olives
- 2 plum tomatoes, chopped
- 1 clove garlic, minced
- 1 cup thinly sliced red onion
- 2 tbsp. chopped fresh parsley
- 1/4 tsp. pepper
- 1/4 tsp. salt
- 2 tbsp. balsamic vinegar

Directions

Put spinach in a bowl.

Add oil to a skillet set over medium heat; add onion and sauté, stirring, for about 2 minutes or until tender. Stir in garlic, parsley, olives and tomatoes and cook, stirring for about 3 minutes or until tomatoes break down. Stir in vinegar, beets, salt and pepper and continue cooking for 1 more minute or until the beets are heated through. Toss together spinach and beet mixture until well blended. Serve warm.

Citrus and Spinach Salad

Yields: 4 Servings

Total Time: 15 Minutes

Prep Time: 15 Minutes

Cook Time: N/A

Ingredients

- 2 tbsp. freshly squeezed orange or grapefruit juice
- 1 tsp. poppy seeds
- 8 cups chopped spinach
- 1 clove garlic, very finely chopped
- 1/2 small red onion, thinly sliced
- 1/2 tsp. honey
- 1/2 tbsp. coarse-grain mustard
- 1 tbsp. extra-virgin olive oil
- 1 tbsp. white-wine vinegar
- 1/4 tsp. salt
- Pepper

Directions

Soak onion in a bowl of water for at least 10 minutes; drain and set aside.

In a salad bowl, combine orange (grapefruit) juice, garlic, honey, mustard, extra virgin olive oil, vinegar, salt and pepper; stir in onion, spinach and fruit sections. Serve garnished with poppy seeds.

Superfood Sushi

Yields: 4 Rolls

Total Time: 35 Minutes

Prep Time: 35 Minutes

Cook Time: 0 Minutes

Ingredients

Sushi

- 4 Nori sheets
- 4 asparagus spears, tried and cut into 1/4's , and marinated in tamari
- 1/2 small red bell pepper, julienned
- 1 inch piece fresh ginger, grated
- 1 carrot, julienned
- 1/4 cucumber, julienned, and wet center removed
- 1/2 red or green chili, finely chopped

Cauliflower Rice

- 1/4 of a large cauliflower
- 1 tsp. coconut oil, melted
- 1/4 cup (60 grams) of ground cashew nuts, optional
- 1-2 tsp. rice vinegar
- Sea salt

Directions

Cauliflower Rice:

Grind the cauliflower in a food processor or grate finely. Put in a bowl and toss with a little (1 teaspoon) melted coconut oil. Add the other ingredients and mix well.

Wasabi sauce

- 1 large soft avocado
- 1 teaspoon of wasabi paste
- 1 teaspoon lemon juice
- A little water to required thickness (thin enough to drop off spoon)
- Sea salt and cracked black pepper, optional

Mix all ingredients until smooth

Making the sushi roll

Take a sushi rolling mat, place the Nori sheet shiny side down Spoon enough of the rice onto the sheet and smooth out to make an even layer, leave a 2cm gap at the top and bottom Place thin strips of the vegetables across the sheets, placing the fillings tightly next to each other and slightly on top of each other. Drizzle a line of the wasabi avocado sauce on top of the vegetables

Pick up the near side of the mat and roll the sheet on to itself, with your hands on the mat pull back to yourself to form a tube, move your fingers along to make a firm tube. Take the near side end of the mat and roll it away from yourself. Stick the far side edge to the roll using small amount of water, dip fingers in a bowl and lightly wet the edge. Roll the roll onto and leave for a few seconds. Take a very sharp knife and cut off the ends, about 4cm from the end. Cut into about 6 equal pieces

Serve with my Asian cucumber salad.

Carrot and Goji Berry Soup

Yield: 4 to 6 Servings

Total Time: 55 Minutes

Prep Time: 20 Minutes

Cook Time: 35 Minutes

Ingredients

- 1 ¼ cups fresh carrot juice
- 1 inch ginger, juiced with carrots
- ½ inch turmeric, juiced with carrots
- 1 cup carrots
- 1 cup pumpkin
- 2 tbsp. Goji berries
- 2 tbsp. coconut oil
- 1 cup onion, chopped
- 1 red jalapeno pepper-seeds removed
- 2 cups water
- ½ cup light coconut milk
- 1 clove garlic
- Sea salt and cracked black pepper to taste

Directions

Juice 1 ¼ cups worth of carrots with the turmeric and ginger. Once done, soak the goji berries in the juice for roughly 20 minutes.

Heat coconut oil in a pot and add the onions; sauté for about 4 minutes or until soft, and then add the jalapeno pepper and garlic cook for 1 minute more. Stir in the chopped carrots and water and bring to a boil. Once boiling, reduce heat to a simmer and cook, covered, for about 20 minutes. Cool slightly and transfer the mixture to the blender and add the coconut milk; blend to a thick puree. Strain the goji berries from the carrot juice and set aside.

Add this juice to the puree and continue pureeing until smooth. Season with salt and pepper to taste.

To serve, garnish each serving with of the goji berries.

Cleansing Detox Soup

Yield: 4 Servings

Total Time: 30 Minutes

Prep Time: 10 Minutes

Cook time: 20 Minutes

Ingredients

- 1/4 cup water
- 2 cloves garlic, minced
- 1/2 of a red onion, diced
- 1 tbsp. fresh ginger, peeled and minced
- 1 cup chopped tomatoes
- 1 small head of broccoli, florets
- 3 medium carrots, diced
- 3 celery stalks, diced
- 6 cups water
- 1/4 tsp. cinnamon
- 1 tsp. turmeric
- 1/8 tsp. cayenne pepper
- Sea salt
- Freshly ground black pepper
- juice of 1 lemon
- 1 cup purple cabbage, chopped
- 2 cups kale, torn in pieces

Directions

Bring a large pot of water to a gentle boil over medium heat. Add garlic and onion and cook for about 2 minutes, stirring occasionally. Stir in fresh ginger, tomatoes, broccoli, carrots, and celery and continue cooking for 3 minutes more. Stir in cinnamon, turmeric, cayenne pepper, sea salt and black pepper.

Add in ½ cup water and bring the mixture to a rolling boil; reduce heat and simmer for about 15 minutes or until the veggies and tender. Stir in lemon juice, cabbage, and kale during the last 2 minutes of cooking. Serve hot or warm.

Green Super Detox Salad

Yield: 2 Servings

Total Time: 10 Minutes

Prep Time: 10 Minutes

Cook time: N/A

Ingredients

- 1 tbsp. extra virgin olive oil
- juice from 1 lemon
- 1/2 avocado
- 2 large cucumbers
- 1/4 cabbage
- 1/4 cup chopped celery
- 1/8 cup pistachios
- 1/4 head broccoli
- Sea salt and pepper

Directions

In a large bowl, combine extra virgin olive oil, lemon juice and avocado; mash with a fork until smooth; season with salt and pepper and set aside.

Using a spiralizer or a veggie peeler, make the cucumber noodles.

Chop the remaining ingredients and toss them in a bowl with the cucumber noodles; add the avocado dressing and toss to combine well. Enjoy!

Chilled Green Goddess Soup

Yield: 6 Servings

Total Time: 15 Minutes

Prep Time: 15 Minutes

Cook Time: 0 Minutes

Ingredients

- 6 cups cucumber
- 2 stalks celery chopped
- 1-2 cups water (depending how thin you want it)
- 2 tablespoons fresh lime juice
- 1 cup watercress leaves
- 1 cup rocket leaves
- ½ cup mashed avocado (roughly 1 avocado)
- 1 tsp. wheatgrass power or a mixed green powder, optional
- Sea salt to taste

Directions

Blend all ingredients except the avocado in a blender until a broth forms. Strain the liquid through a cheesecloth or fine sieve. Then return to blender and add the avocado and blend until smooth.

Garnish with a few watercress leaves and cracked black pepper.

Salad For Glowing Skin + Detox Dressing

Yield: 4 Servings

Total Time: 20 Minutes

Prep Time: 20 Minutes

Cook Time: N/A

Ingredients

For the salad:

- 3 ounces organic baby arugula
- 1 small bunch green onions, thinly sliced
- ½ cucumber, thinly sliced
- ½ medium beet, thinly shredded
- 1 large carrot, shredded
- 1 firm ripe avocado, diced
- 2 tbsp. raw sliced almonds
- 2 tbsp. raw pumpkin seeds
- 2 tbsp. sunflower seeds

For the detox dressing:

- ½ tsp. raw honey
- Juice of 2 lemons
- ½ cup avocado oil
- Pinch sea salt
- Pinch dry mustard powder
- Pinch black pepper
- ¼ cup freshly chopped parsley

Directions

Make the salad: Toss arugula with sliced and shredded veggies in a large bowl. Sprinkle with seeds and nuts and set aside.

Make the Dressing: Combine honey and lemon juice in a jar with a tight fitting lid; shake until honey is dissolved. Add avocado oil, salt, mustard powder, and pepper and fit the lid; shake vigorously until well blended. Add parsley and continue shaking to mix well. Pour the dressing over the salad and toss to coat well. Serve immediately.

Cauliflower Couscous Salad

Yield: 4 Servings

Total Time: 25 Minutes

Prep Time: 25 Minutes

Cook Time: N/A

Ingredients

- 1 large head cauliflower, cut into florets
- 3-4 green onions, thinly sliced
- 2 garlic cloves, finely minced
- 1 jalapeño, seeds and ribs removed, minced
- 1 cup shredded carrots
- 1 cup diced celery
- 1 cup diced cucumber
- 1 green apple, diced
- Juice of 1 lemon
- 1 tbsp. extra-virgin olive oil
- Sea salt
- Freshly ground black pepper

Directions

Working in two batches, pulse cauliflower florets in a food processor until finely chopped.

Transfer to a bowl and add the remaining ingredients; toss until well combined. Serve immediately.

Broccoli Detox Soup

Yield: 2 Servings

Total Time: 20 Minutes

Prep Time: 5 Minutes

Cook Time: 15 Minutes

Ingredients

- 1 tsp. coconut oil
- 2 garlic cloves, crushed
- 1 onion, diced
- 2 cups broccoli florets
- 1 carrot, chopped
- 1 parsnip, chopped
- 2 celery stalks, diced
- 2 cups filtered water
- 1 cup greens (beet greens, spinach, kale, or any other available)
- Juice of ½ lemon
- 1 tbsp. chia seeds
- ½ tsp. sea salt
- 1 tsp. coconut milk, to serve
- Toasted mixed seeds and nuts, to serve

Directions

Heat coconut oil in a soup pot set over low heat; stir in garlic, onion, broccoli, celery sticks, parsnip, and carrot; cook for about 5 minutes, stirring frequently.

Stir in water and bring the mixture to a gentle boil; cover and simmer for about 7 minutes or until veggies are tender.

Stir in the greens and transfer to a food processor or blender; add lemon juice, chia seeds, and sea salt and pulse until very smooth.

Stir in coconut milk and sprinkle with toasted seeds and serve right away.

Roasted Power Bowl w/ Lemon Tahini Dressing

Yield: 8 Servings

Total Time: 25 Minutes

Prep Time: 10 Minutes

Cook time: 15 Minutes

Ingredients

- 1½ pounds sweet potatoes, diced
- 3 tbsp. olive oil, divided
- 1 tsp. kosher salt, divided
- 1 head cauliflower, cut into florets
- Fresh ground pepper
- 1 to 1 ½ cups quinoa
- 15-ounce can chickpeas (1½ cups cooked),drained and rinsed
- 1 beet, thinly sliced
- ⅓ cup sunflower seeds
- 12 cups salad greens
- ¼ head red cabbage (you can combine savoy and red), thinly sliced

Lemon Tahini Dressing

- 1 tbsp. extra-virgin olive oil
- ½ cup freshly squeezed lemon juice
- ½ cup tahini
- ½ tsp. kosher salt

Directions

Preheat your oven to 450°F.

Place sweet potatoes in a large bowl, add 1 ½ tablespoons of extra virgin olive oil and ½ teaspoon of sea salt; toss to coat well.

Transfer the sweet potatoes to a parchment paper lined baking sheet, pushing them onto one half of the sheet. Pour cauliflower florets onto the other half of the sheet and sprinkle with pepper; roast for about 30 minutes or until tender.

In the meantime, follow package instructions to prepare quinoa.

In a bowl, mix chickpeas with a drizzle of extra virgin olive oil and sea salt.

Peel and thinly slice the beet. Thinly slice the red cabbage.

Make the dressing:

Combine extra virgin olive oil, lemon juice, tahini, and salt in a small bowl; whisk to combine well.

Divide the salad greens among the four serving bowls and top each with small piles of each component. Pour the dressing over each serving and scatter with sunflower seeds.

Lemony Asparagus & Tomato Salad

Yield: 2-3 Servings

Total Time: 5 Minutes

Prep Time: 5 Minutes

Cook Time: N/A

Ingredients

- 1 pint cherry tomatoes, halved
- 1 large bunch of asparagus, thinly sliced
- Juice of 1 lemon
- 3 tbsp. extra virgin olive oil
- Sea salt and black pepper
- 2 tbsp. freshly chopped parsley

Directions

In a medium bowl, combine tomatoes and asparagus.

In a small bowl, whisk together lemon juice, extra virgin olive oil, sea salt and pepper; pour the dressing over the salad and toss to coat well. Top with parsley and enjoy!

Kale Avocado Salad with Orange

Yield: 2 Servings

Total Time: 10 Minutes

Prep Time: 10 Minutes

Cook Time: N/A

Ingredients

Salad

- 2-3 handfuls kale, rinsed and chopped
- ½ cup green peas
- ½ avocado, sliced
- ½ cucumber, sliced
- 1 orange, sliced
- 2 tbsp. almond slices
- 2 tbsp. hemp seeds, shelled

Vinaigrette

- 2 tbsp. extra virgin olive oil
- 3 tbsp. fresh lemon juice
- Pinch garlic powder
- Sea salt
- Black pepper

Directions

Place chopped kale in a bowl. In a small bowl, whisk together extra virgin olive oil, lemon juice, garlic powder, sea salt and pepper; using your hands, massage the lemon vinaigrette into the kale for about 2 minutes or until kale begins to soften.

Divide the between two serving plates and add peas, avocado, cucumber, and orange slices.

Top with almond slices and hemp seeds; drizzle with lemon juice and sprinkle with cracked pepper. Enjoy!

Healthy Detox Soup

Yield: 4 Servings

Total Time: 48 Minutes

Prep Time: 10 Minutes

Cook time: 38 Minutes

Ingredients:

- 4 cloves garlic, crushed
- 2 medium leeks, chopped
- 1 serrano pepper, thinly sliced
- 4 celery stalks, chopped
- 4 carrots, diced
- 3 rutabagas, peeled and diced
- 8 cups water
- 2 cups pinto beans, cooked with cooking liquids
- 3 tomatoes, diced
- 3 zucchini, diced
- 2 bunches kale, thinly sliced
- 3 tablespoons lemon juice
- Sea salt
- Freshly cracked black pepper

Directions

Heat a pot over medium heat; add garlic, leeks, and serranos. Cook for about 5 minutes, stirring. Add celery, carrots, and rutabagas; cook for about 3 minutes more and stir in water, pinto beans, and tomatoes; simmer for about 30 minutes or until the beans are cooked through. Stir in zucchini and kale, 15 minutes before serving. Remove from heat and stir in lemon juice; season with sea salt and black pepper and serve.

The Ultimate Kale Salad

Yield: 4 Servings

Total Time: 10 Minutes

Prep Time: 10 Minutes

Cook time: N/A

Ingredients

- 1 head kale, rinsed and finely chopped into strips
- ¼ white cabbage, thinly sliced
- 1 handful pumpkin seeds
- 1 spring onion, chopped
- 2 sundried tomatoes, chopped

For the dressing

- 50g almond butter
- 1 tbsp. ground nut oil
- 1 tbsp. tamari
- Juice 1 lime
- Pinch sea salt

Directions

Place the kale into a large bowl, add cabbage, pumpkin seeds, spring onions and sundried tomatoes.

Make the dressing: Combine all dressing in a bowl and mix until well blended.

Pour the dressing over the salad and massage thoroughly with your hands to blend flavors.

Serve and enjoy.

Chickpea Salad w/ Zucchini & Avocado Mayo

Yield: 4 Servings

Total Time: 2 Hours 20 Minutes

Prep Time: 20 Minutes

Cook time: 2 Hours

Ingredients

- 100g chickpeas
- Juice ½ lemon
- 1 teaspoon rapeseed oil
- 4 chives, chopped
- Handful parsley, chopped
- 100g cherry tomatoes, halved
- 5 radishes, chopped
- 2 spring onions, sliced
- Handful cashew nuts, toasted
- Pinch sea salt
- Pinch black pepper
- 1 yellow zucchini, cut into strips

For the avocado mayonnaise

- 1/2 avocado
- 3 chives, chopped
- Juice ½ lemon
- 1 teaspoon rapeseed oil
- Pinch sea salt
- Pinch black pepper

Directions

Soak the chickpeas in water for at least 8 hours or overnight.

When ready to use, drain the chickpeas and transfer to a pan. Cover with double the amount of water and bring to a rolling boil. Lower heat and simmer for about 2hours or until tender; drain and let cool.

Transfer the cooked chickpeas to a bowl and stir in lemon juice, rapeseed oil, chives, parsley, tomatoes, radishes, spring onions, toasted cashew nuts, sea salt and pepper; set aside.

Make the mayonnaise: In a food processor, combine avocado, chives, lemon juice, oil, sea salt and pepper; pulse until you achieve the consistency of mayonnaise. Transfer the avocado mayo to a bowl and mix in the yellow zucchini.

Place the zucchini in a bowl and top with chickpea salad; add a dollop of avocado mayo and garnish with fresh chili. Enjoy!

Whole Food Dinner Recipes

Shrimp Salad w/ Grapefruit and Avocado

Yield: 2 Servings

Total Time: 20 Minutes

Prep Time: 10 Minutes

Cook Time: 10 Minutes

Ingredients

- 2 tbsp. chili oil
- 1 cup shrimp
- ½ tsp. salt
- ½ tsp. pepper
- 1 avocado, cubed
- 1 grapefruit, cubed
- ¼ cup lemon juice

Directions

Heat chili oil in a saucepan set over medium heat; add shrimp and cook until opaque and lightly browned.

Remove the pan from heat and season shrimp with sea salt and pepper.

In a serving bowl, pack avocado slices as tightly as possible, and then top with a layer of shrimp, grapefruit, and drizzle with lemon juice. Serve while shrimp are still hot!

Orange-Cranberry Crusted Salmon

Yield: 4 Servings

Total Time: 35 Minutes

Prep Time: 15 Minutes

Cook time: 20 Minutes

Ingredients

- Olive oil cooking spray
- 4 salmon filets
- Salt & pepper to taste
- 2 tbsp. extra virgin olive oil
- ¼ cup dried cranberries, chopped
- ½ cup walnuts, chopped
- 1 tsp. orange zest
- 1 tbsp. Dijon mustard
- 2 tbsp. parsley, chopped

Directions

Preheat your oven to 370°F. Lightly coat a baking sheet with olive oil cooking spray. Generously season the fish filets with sea salt and pepper and arrange them on the baking sheet.

Mix the remaining ingredients in a small bowl until well blended; press onto the filets and bake in the reheated oven for about 20 minutes or until the topping is lightly browned.

Remove from oven and serve.

Turkey & Quinoa Salad

Yield: 4 Servings

Total Time: 40 Minutes

Prep Time: 20 Minutes

Cook Time: 20 Minutes

Ingredients

- 3 tbsp. extra-virgin olive oil
- 1 1/2 cups quinoa, rinsed
- Kosher salt
- 1 pound turkey cutlets
- 3 tbsp. chopped fresh tarragon and/or parsley
- Freshly ground pepper
- 1/2 small red onion, halved and sliced
- 1 1/2 pounds assorted heirloom tomatoes, chopped
- 1 chile pepper, seeded and chopped
- 4 cucumbers, chopped
- 2 tbsp. sherry vinegar

Directions

In a large skillet set over medium high heat, heat ½ tablespoon of extra virgin olive oil; stir in quinoa and cook, stirring continuously for about 4minutes or until lightly toasted. Stir in salt and 4 cups of water; bring to a gentle boil, lower heat and simmer for about 15 minutes.

In a mixing bowl, toss together turkey, half of herbs, a pinch of sea salt and pepper; set aside.

In a bowl, soak the sliced onion in cold water for at least 10 minutes.

In a separate bowl, toss together, cucumbers, chile, tomatoes, the remaining herbs,1 ½ tablespoons extra virgin olive oil, vinegar, sea salt and black pepper.

Drain onion and stir into the tomato mixture.

Heat the remaining 1 tablespoon olive oil in a large nonstick skillet over medium-high heat. Working in batches, add the turkey and cook until golden, about 3 minutes per side. Drain on paper towels, then cut into 2-inch pieces. Fluff the quinoa with a fork and divide among bowls. Top with the tomato mixture and turkey.

Salmon Salad

Yield: 2 Servings

Total Time: 15 Minutes

Prep Time: 5 Minutes

Cook Time: 10 Minutes

Ingredients

- 7 ounces wild caught salmon fillets, skinned
- 7 ounces broccoli
- 1 tbsp. extra virgin olive oil
- 2 spring onions, thinly sliced
- ½ red chilli, deseeded, chopped
- 1 tbsp. mixed seeds (sesame seeds, sunflower seeds, pumpkin seeds, and linseeds)
- 1/8 cup chopped nuts (almonds or brazil nuts)
- Juice of 1 orange
- 1 orange, zested

Directions

In a skillet, bring water to a gentle boil. Add fish and broccoli and cook 3 minutes or until fish is cooked through and broccoli is tender.

Remove from heat and let cool a bit; drain the broccoli and set aside.

Heat extra virgin olive oil in a pan; add onions, chilli, seeds and nuts and fry for about 4 minutes or until golden.

Stir in orange juice and zest and season with sea salt and cracked black pepper.

Flake the fish into small pieces and mix with broccoli. Serve topped with nut and chilli mixture.

Flake the salmon into pieces, mix with the broccoli and sprinkle the chilli and nut mixture over the top.

Lemongrass and Chilli Beef

Yield: 4 Serving

Total Time: 40 Minutes

Prep Time: 15 Minutes

Cook time: 25 Minutes

Ingredients

- 3.5 ounces zucchini noodles
- 4 ounces extra-lean beef steak, trimmed, sliced
- 1/2 tbsp. sunflower oil
- 1 tsp. fish sauce
- Juice of 1 lime
- 1 tsp. honey
- 1 garlic clove
- ½ piece ginger, chopped
- 1 lemongrass stem, chopped
- 1 red chilli, chopped
- 1/2 cup each mint, basil and coriander
- 1 spring onions, sliced

Directions

In a food processor, process together garlic, ginger, lemongrass and chilli into a paste. Add a tablespoon oil, fish sauce, lime juice and palm sugar and process until well combined.

Toss meat in a large bowl with half marinade and chill for at least 15 minutes.

In the meantime, cook zucchini noodles; drain and rinse under cold water.

Toss vermicelli with the remaining marinade.

Add oil to a pan set over medium high heat; add beef and cook for about 7 minutes or until browned.

Toss together rice noodles, herbs and onions in a bowl; serve topped with beef.

Liver and Onions

Yield: 4 Serving

Total Time: 21 Minutes

Prep Time: 15 Minutes

Cook time: 6 Minutes

Ingredients

- 2 tbsp. extra virgin olive oil
- 5 large onions, sliced;
- 4 large slices beef liver;
- Salt
- Pepper

Directions

Add olive oil to a skillet set over medium low heat; sauté onions until tender and caramelized.

Place liver to a separate pan set over medium high heat and cook for about 3 minutes per side or until cooked through.

Top the liver with the caramelized onions and homemade salsa.

Shrimp & Zucchini w/ Herbed Quinoa

Yield: 1 Serving

Total Time: 40Minutes

Prep Time: 15 Minutes

Cook time: 25 Minutes

Ingredients

- 1 cup water
- 2/3 cup (150 grams) quinoa
- 1 tbsp. extra virgin olive oil
- 1 garlic clove, minced
- 1 1/2 cups thinly sliced zucchini
- 3 ounces cooked shrimp
- 1/4 cup thinly chopped fresh chives and basil
- Juice of1 lemon

Directions

Combine water and quinoa in a skillet; bring to a gentle boil, cover and simmer for about 15 minutes or until all the water is absorbed.

In a pan, heat extra virgin olive oil; add garlic and sauté for about 2 minutes or until fragrant. Add zucchini and cook for about 6 minutes or until tender. Stir in shrimp and cook for 3 minutes more or until warmed through.

Using a fork, fluff the cooked quinoa and toss with shrimp, zucchini and fresh herbs. Serve, drizzled with fresh lemon juice.

Cajun Chicken w/ Detox Salad & Mango Salsa

Yield: 4 Servings

Total Time: 32 Minutes

Prep Time: 20 Minutes

Cook time: 12 Minutes

Ingredients

- 1 tsp. extra virgin olive oil
- 1 garlic clove, crushed
- 1 tsp. crushed dried chilli
- 1 tbsp. ground coriander
- 2 tbsp. ground cumin
- 1 tbsp. smoked paprika
- 4 (159 gram each) chicken breasts, boneless, skinless

For the salad

- 1 tbsp. rapeseed oil
- 150g spinach, chopped
- 1/4 red onion, roughly diced
- A handful fresh parsley
- A handful fresh coriander
- A handful fresh mint
- 2 avocados, sliced

For the mango salsa

- 4 cherry tomatoes, diced
- 1 mango, diced
- 1 fresh red chilli, seeded and finely chopped
- Juice of 1 lime
- A handful of fresh coriander, finely chopped
- Sea salt
- Black pepper

Directions

Make the marinade: In a large bowl, mix together extra virgin olive oil, garlic, all spices, and salt .Add the chicken and turn until well coated with the marinade.

Heat a grill pan or griddle over medium heat.

In the meantime, working with one at a time, transfer the chicken breasts on side of a large cling film sheet and fold over to seal in the spices; with a rolling pin, gently bash the chicken until flatten to about 1 cm thick. Transfer the chicken breasts to a griddle pan and cook over medium heat for about 6 minutes per side or until cooked through.

Make the salad: In a large mixing bowl, mix rapeseed oil, spinach, red onion, parsley, mint, and coriander. Gently fold in avocado slices and season with sea salt and black pepper.

Make salsa: In a separate bowl, mix together all the salsa ingredients; with your hands, squeeze the tomatoes until a chunky, juicy salsa is formed.

Serve one chicken breast with a heaping of spinach salad, topped with mango salsa.

Shrimp Fried Cauliflower Rice

Yield: 4 Servings

Total Time: 20 Minutes

Prep Time: 15 Minutes

Cook Time: 5 Minutes

Ingredients

- 2 eggs, beaten
- 2 cups cooked cauliflower rice
- 1/4 cup chopped red bell pepper
- 1/2 cup peas
- 1 medium carrot, chopped
- 8 oz. peeled and deveined shrimp
- 2 cloves garlic, minced
- 1 cup chopped onion
- 1 tbsp. coconut oil
- Salt
- Pepper

Directions

Melt coconut oil in a pan set over medium high heat; add garlic and onion and sauté for about 4 minutes or until tender. Stir in shrimp for about 1 minute.

Stir in bell pepper, peas, and carrot and cook for about 4 minutes. Stir in cauliflower rice and make a well in the center of the mixture. Pour the beaten eggs in the well and stir to scramble. Season with salt and pepper to serve.

Fried Salmon Fillets

Yield: 3 Servings

Total Time: 35 Minutes

Prep Time: 15 Minutes

Cook Time: 20 Minutes

Ingredients

- 5 ounces tilapia fillet, skin and bones removed
- ¼ tsp. basil
- ¼ tsp. ground paprika
- ¼ tsp. oregano
- ¼ tsp. ground white pepper
- ¼ tsp. thyme
- ¼ tsp. ground black pepper
- 2 tsp. salt
- ¼ tsp. onion powder
- ¼ tsp. ground cayenne pepper
- 2 tsp. extra virgin olive oil
- ¼ cup cooked brown rice, for serving

Directions

Combine oregano, basil, thyme, black pepper, white pepper, salt, onion powder, cayenne pepper, and paprika in a small bowl.

Brush fish with half of oil and sprinkle with the spice mixture. Drizzle with the remaining oil and cook fish in a skillet set over

high heat until blackened and flakes easily with a fork. Serve
with cooked brown rice.

Chicken w/Peppers

Yield: 2 Servings

Total Time: 40 Minutes

Prep Time: 15 Minutes

Cook Time: 25 Minutes

Ingredients

- 2 tsp. extra virgin olive oil

- 10 ounces chicken breast halves, skinless, boneless, trimmed

- 3 kalamata olives

- ¼ cups tomato, chopped

- ¼ red bell pepper, cut into small strips

- ¼ yellow bell pepper, cut into small strips

- ¼ cups onion, sliced

- Cooking spray

- 1 tsp. oregano, chopped

- ½ tbsp. parsley, chopped

- ¼ tsp. pepper

- ¼ tsp. salt

Directions

In a nonstick skillet, sauté onion in oil over medium high heat for about 5 minutes or until golden brown. Raise heat to high and stir in bell peppers; sauté until peppers are tender, for about 10 minutes. Stir in tomato, black pepper and salt and continue cooking for 7 more minutes or until all liquid has evaporated. Stir in olives, oregano, and parsley and cook for 1 more minute. Transfer the mixture to a bowl and keep warm.

Wipe the pan clean and coat it lightly with cooking spray. Add chicken and cook until done, for about 3 minutes per side. Stir in the tomato mixture and cook until heated through, for about 1 minute.

Vegetarian Curry

Yield: 2 servings

Total Time: 45 minutes

Prep Time: 15 minutes

Cook Time: 30 minutes

- 2 tbsp. coconut oil
- 1 large yellow onion, finely diced
- 4 medium cloves garlic, minced
- 1 tbsp. grated fresh ginger
- 1 tbsp. ground coriander
- 1 tbsp. ground cumin
- 1 sp. ground turmeric
- 1/2 tsp. cayenne
- 2 tbsp. tomato paste
- 3 cups vegetable broth
- 1 cup light coconut milk
- One 3-inch cinnamon stick
- Fine sea salt and freshly ground black pepper
- 4 cups cauliflower florets
- 3 cups sweet potatoes chunks
- 1 ½ cups chopped tomatoes
- 1 cup carrots chunks
- 2 zucchini, cut into 1/2 inch chunks
- 1 15-1/2-ounce can chickpeas, drained and rinsed
- ½ cup baby spinach
- 3 tbsp. fresh lime juice
- 2 tsp. finely grated lime zest
- 3 tbsp. chopped fresh cilantro

Directions

Heat oil in a heavy-duty pot over medium high heat; stir in onion for about 3 minutes or until browned.

Lower heat to medium and stir in ginger and garlic; cook, stirring, for about 1 minute or until flavors blend. Stir in turmeric, cumin, coriander, and cayenne and cook for about 1 minute. Stir in tomato paste and cock for 1 minute more.

Add coconut milk, broth, cinnamon, salt, and pepper; bring the curry to a gentle boil. Lower heat and simmer for about 10 minutes.

Stir in carrots, tomatoes, sweet potatoes and cauliflower; returnto a boil and simmer for about 20 minutes or until the veggies are tender.

Stir in lime juice, zest, zucchini, spinach, and chickpeas and cook for about 5 minutes or until spinach is wilted.

Warm Lemon Chicken

Yield: 2 Servings

Total Time: 30 Minutes

Prep Time: 15 Minutes

Cook Time: 15 Minutes

Ingredients

- 10 ounces chicken thighs, skinless, boneless
- ½ red cabbage, shredded
- 20g baby spinach leaves
- 1 tsp. balsamic vinegar
- 1 carrots, cut into ribbons
- ½ tsp. extra virgin olive oil
- 1 sprig thyme
- Juice and zest from 1/2 lemons
- 1 crushed garlic cloves

Directions

Remove the skin from the chicken and place it between two baking sheets; bash with a meat tenderizer or a rolling pin to flatten.

Place the chicken in a dish and generously season with pepper and salt. Stir in half lemon juice and lemon zest and sprinkle with thyme.

Set a pan or griddle over medium heat and fry the chicken for about 15 minutes or until cooked through and golden brown.

In a bowl, combine carrots, red cabbage and spinach. Divide salad between serving plates and top each with chicken. Drizzle with the remaining lemon juice, balsamic vinegar and cooking juices.

Cauliflower Pizza

Yield: 2 Servings

Total Time: 45 Minutes

Prep Time: 15 Minutes

Cook Time: 30 Minutes

Ingredients for the base:

- ½ head (400 grams) cauliflower florets
- 1 egg
- 1 tsp. chopped rosemary
- 1 tsp. chopped thyme
- Pinch of Cayenne Pepper
- Salt and freshly ground black pepper to taste

Ingredients for topping: (You can be as inventive as you like! Use whatever you wish.)

Examples:

- Homemade vegan Pesto
- Sun Blushed Tomatoes

Directions:

Pre-heat your oven to 400F. Chop the cauliflower into little florets and then blend in food processor until it looks like flour. You then want to steam the 'flour' for about 5 minutes. Once you have steamed the cauliflower, place it in a muslin cloth or a clean tea towel and string out all the water.

There will be a lot, so you want to make sure you get as much out as possible!

Next, you want to take your cauliflower and all in your egg and seasoning of choice. Make sure the cauliflower is cool before adding the egg. Mix together with your hands, and it should be almost dough-like!

With your dough roll out on to a baking dish, into a shape of your choice... round, rectangle or even heart! Place in the oven and cook for roughly 30 minutes or until golden. Remove and place on your toppings. Put it back in the oven for a further 10 minutes.

Take out, and enjoy your guilt-free pizza!

Warm Lemon Chicken

Yield: 4 Servings

Total Time: 30 Minutes

Prep Time: 15 Minutes

Cook time: 15 Minutes

Ingredients

- 10 ounces chicken thighs, skinless, boneless
- ½ red cabbage, shredded
- 20g baby spinach leaves
- 1 tsp. balsamic vinegar
- 1 carrots, cut into ribbons
- ½ tsp. extra virgin olive oil
- 1 sprig thyme
- Juice and zest from 1/2 lemons
- 1 crushed garlic cloves

Directions

Remove the skin from the chicken and place it between two baking sheets; bash with a meat tenderizer or a rolling pin to flatten.

Place the chicken in a dish and generously season with pepper and salt. Stir in half lemon juice and lemon zest and sprinkle with thyme.

Set a pan or griddle over medium heat and fry the chicken for about 15 minutes or until cooked through and golden brown.

In a bowl, combine carrots, red cabbage and spinach. Divide salad between serving plates and top each with chicken. Drizzle with the remaining lemon juice, balsamic vinegar and cooking juices.

Coconut Chicken

Yield: 4 Servings

Total Time: 25 Minutes

Prep Time: 15 Minutes

Cook time: 10 Minutes

Ingredients

- 8 ounces chicken breast, boneless, skinless
- ½ tsp. coconut oil
- 3 egg whites
- 1 tsp. sea salt
- 1 tbsp. coconut, shredded
- 1 tbsp. whole-wheat flour

Directions

In a bowl, combine shredded coconut, flour and sea salt.

In a separate bowl, beat the egg; dip the chicken in the egg and roll in the flour mixture until well coated.

Add coconut oil to a pan set over medium heat and fry the chicken until the crust begins to brown.

Transfer the chicken to the oven and bake at 350°F for about 10 minutes.

Chicken Bruschetta

Yield: 4 Servings

Total Time: 25 Minutes

Prep Time: 15 Minutes

Cook time: 10 Minutes

Ingredients

- 10 ounces chicken breasts, skinless, boneless
- ½ tsp. extra virgin olive oil
- 1.8 ounces cherry tomatoes
- 1 tsp. white vinegar
- 0.5 ounces fresh basil leaves
- 1 small cloves garlic, minced
- 1 small onions, chopped

Directions

Add half of the oil to the skillet and cook chicken over medium heat.

In the meantime, slice basil leaves and prepare the veggies.

Heat the remaining oil and sauté garlic and onion for about 3 minutes. Stir in basil and tomatoes for about 5 minutes. Stir in vinegar.

Serve the cooked chicken; cook until heated through and serve topped with onion and tomato mixture.

Beetroot and Carrot Burgers

Yield: 8 (90g/3.2 ounces) burgers

Total Time: 1Hour 30 Minutes

Prep Time: 30 Minutes

Cook Time: 1 Hour

Ingredients:

- 1 cup grated beetroot
- 1 cup grated carrot
- 100g oatmeal
- 3 Eggs (or you can substitute with flax 'eggs')
- 1 Shallot finely chopped
- 6 tbsp. chopped dill/parsley or any herbs
- Oil (for frying), I use coconut oil
- 8 portobello mushrooms
- 2 cups (450 grams) fresh spinach
- 1 garlic clove
- 1 pinch of cayenne
- 1 tbsp. hemp seeds

Instructions

Before mixing the ingredients together, make sure you have squeezed out some of the liquid from the beetroot and carrot. (This is a perfect carrot/ beetroot juice to have whilst cooking!). Then beat together eggs, oatmeal, carrot, beetroot, dill, hemp seeds, shallot, and parsley in a bowl until well blended. Season with salt and cayenne pepper and press the mixture together form a ball, cover and keep chilled in the fridge for 1 hour, or longer.

Pre-heat the oven to 350F. Then divide your mixture into roughly 8 burgers (around 90g each). Roll each ball together and then flatten slightly.

In a pan, heat a little oil and once hot, fry the burgers until each side is sealed and browned (about 2 minutes per side). Place on a baking sheet and bake at the same time as the mushrooms. In a separate pan cook the garlic with some oil until soft. Pour this mixture evenly on each of the mushrooms, and then bake upright.

Cook burgers and mushrooms in the oven for 20-25 minutes.

To wilt the spinach either cook briefly in hot water or in pan with a little oil. Or just put raw on top of the mushroom before serving with the beet root.

Serve alongside the burgers with a tomato chutney or sweet chili jam!

Whole Food Snacks

Vegan Beet Burgers

Yield: 4 Servings

Total Time: 45 Minutes

Prep Time: 15 Minutes

Cook time: 30 Minutes

Ingredients

- 3/4 cup of water
- 1/4 cup ground flax seeds
- 3 carrots
- 1 medium beet
- 3 stalks of kale
- 1/2 bunch of parsley
- 1 tsp. onion powder
- 1 tsp. garlic powder
- ¼ cup plus 2 tablespoons gluten-free mustard
- 1 tsp. cayenne pepper
- 1 tsp. sea salt
- ½ cup sprouts
- 1 bunch collard leaves

Directions

Preheat your oven to 350°F.

In a bowl, combine water and ground flax; refrigerate until the mixture gels into "flax eggs".

Run the carrots, beet, kale and parsley through a juicer.

Mix the veggie juice with "flax eggs", onion powder, garlic powder, cayenne pepper, sea salt and 2 tablespoons gluten-free mustard.

Form small patties from the mixture and arrange them on a paper-lined baking sheet; bake for about 15 minutes, flip the patties over and bake for 15 minutes more.

Serve each patty inside one collard leaf and top with the remaining gluten-free mustard and sprouts; wrap like a burrito and enjoy!

Spinach Cake

Yields: 12 Cakes

Total Time: 25 Minutes

Prep Time: 15 Minutes

Cook Time: 10 Minutes

Ingredients

- 1 ½ pounds spinach, rinsed
- 2 large eggs, whisked
- 2 cloves garlic, minced
- 1 cup pine nuts
- 3 tbsp. grapeseed oil
- ½ cup currants
- 1 tsp. sea salt

Directions

Wilt spinach in a pan set over low heat for about 5 minutes; drain and let cool a bit before squeezing moisture out of the spinach.

Pulse the spinach in a food processor until coarsely chopped; set aside.

Warm oil in a skillet; add pine nuts and sauté for a few minutes or until golden browned.

Stir in garlic and continue cooking for 1 more minute.

Combine the pine mixture, currants, blended spinach and salt in a bowl; spread the mixture into a coated baking dish and bake at 350°F for about 35 minutes.

Carrot French Fries

Yields: 2 Servings

Total Time: 35 Minutes

Prep Time: 15 Minutes

Cook Time: 20 Minutes

Ingredients

- 2 tbsp. extra virgin olive oil

- 6 large carrots

- ½ tsp. sea salt

Directions

Chop the carrots into 2-inch sections and then cut each section into thin sticks.

Toss together the carrots sticks with extra virgin olive oil and salt in a bowl and spread into a baking sheet lined with parchment paper.

Bake the carrot sticks at 425° for about 20 minutes or until browned.

Roasted Balsamic Beets

Yields: 5 Servings

Total Time: 1 Hour 30 Minutes

Prep Time: 15 Minutes

Cook Time: 1 Hour 15 Minutes

Ingredients

- 2 tbsp. extra virgin olive oil
- 1 tbsp. balsamic vinegar
- 3-4 medium beets
- ½ tsp. sea salt

Directions

Scrub the beets and wash well; cut into 6 wedges and place them in a baking dish.

Drizzle the beets with extra virgin olive oil, vinegar and salt and bake, covered, at 375°F for about 1 hour. Uncover and continue baking for 15 more minutes or until almost tender.

Candied Macadamia Nuts

Yields: 6 Servings

Total Time: 25 Minutes

Prep Time: 10 Minutes

Cook Time: 15 Minutes

Ingredients

- 2 cups macadamia nuts

- 1 tbsp. extra virgin olive oil

- 2 tbsp. agave nectar or honey

- ½ tsp. sea salt

Directions

In a bowl, toss together all ingredients and spread into a baking dish. Bake at 350°F for about 15 minutes or until browned.

Remove from oven and let cool before serving.

Guacamole w/ Vegetables

Yields: 2 Servings

Total Time: 15 Minutes

Prep Time: 15 Minutes

Cook Time: 0 Minutes

Ingredients

- 1 avocado
- Juice of 1 lime
- Zest of lime
- 1 clove garlic, peeled, minced
- 1/4 red onion, peeled, diced
- Fresh cilantro, chopped
- Sea salt
- Veggies (peppers, celery, cucumber etc.) for serving

Directions

In a bowl, mash together all ingredients to your desired consistency. Garnish with cilantro sprigs and store, covered, in a plastic wrap.

Stuffed Mushrooms

Yields: 4 Servings

Total Time: 25 Minutes

Prep Time: 5 Minutes

Cook Time: 10 Minutes

Ingredients

- 1 package (8 ounce) mushrooms
- ¼ cup extra virgin olive oil
- 1 tsp. lemon juice
- 1 clove garlic, chopped
- ½ cup pine nuts
- ½ cup sun dried tomatoes
- 1 cup parsley, chopped
- ¼ tsp. sea salt

Directions

Pulse parsley in a food processor until well chopped.

Add lemon juice, garlic, pine nuts, sundried tomatoes and salt and continue pulsing until smooth.

Add extra virgin olive oil and pulse to blend well.

Remove the stems from mushrooms; stuff each with pesto and bake at 350°F for about 10 minutes.

Squash W/ Cherries

Yields: 8 Servings

Total Time: 25 Minutes

Prep Time: 5 Minutes

Cook Time: 10 Minutes

Ingredients

- 1 large butternut squash, cubed
- 1 cup apple juice
- 10 slivers lemon peel
- 3 cinnamon sticks
- 3 vanilla beans
- ½ cup dried cherries
- ½ tsp. sea salt

Directions

In a baking dish, toss together all the ingredients and bake, covered, at 350°F for about 60 minutes. Uncover and continue baking for 10 more minutes or until browned.

Squash Fries

Yields: 6 Servings

Total Time: 25 Minutes

Prep Time: 15 Minutes

Cook Time: 10 Minutes

Ingredients

- 1 tbsp. grapeseed oil

- 1 medium butternut squash

- 1/8 tsp. sea salt

Directions

Peel and remove seeds from the squash; cut into thin slices and place them in a bowl. Coat with extra virgin olive oil and grapeseed oil; sprinkle with salt and toss to coat well.

Arrange the squash slices onto three baking sheets and broil in the oven until crispy.

Stuffed Celery Bites

Yields: 8 Servings

Total Time: 20 Minutes

Prep Time: 15 Minutes

Cook Time: 5 Minutes

Ingredients:

- Celery leaves

- 2 tbsp. sunflower seeds, dry-roasted

- 1/4 cup Italian cheese blend, shredded

- 1 (8-ounce) fat-free cream cheese

- 8 stalks celery

- 1 clove garlic, minced

- 2 tbsp. pine nuts

- Olive oil cooking spray

Directions:

Coat a nonstick skillet with olive oil cooking spray; add garlic and pine nuts and sauté over medium heat for about 4 minutes or until the nuts are golden brown. Set aside.

Cut off the wide base and tops from celery and remove 2 thin strips from the round side of celery to create a flat surface.

Combine Italian cheese and cream cheese in a bowl; spread into celery and cut each celery stalk into 2-inch pieces.

Sprinkle half of the celery pieces with sunflower seeds and half with the pine nut mixture; cover and let stand for at least 4 hours before serving.

Pesto-Stuffed Mushrooms

Yield: 14 Servings

Total Time: 15 Minutes + Dehydration Time

Prep Time: 15 Minutes

Cook Time: N/A

Ingredients:

- 14+ button mushrooms, washed and stemmed
- 1/2 cup extra virgin olive oil
- 3 cloves garlic
- 2 cups basil
- 1/2 cup pine nuts
- 1 cup walnuts
- 1/2 tsp. sea salt

Directions:

Arrange the mushroom caps top-side down on a plate.

In a food processor, blend together stuffing ingredients until very smooth.

Scoop an equal amount of the stuffing into each cap and dehydrate at 105°F until soft, for about 6 hours.

Serve warm.

Healthy Sautéed Kale

Yields: 4 Servings

Total Time: 35 Minutes

Prep Time: 15 Minutes

Cook Time: 20 Minutes

Ingredients

- 1 bunch kale, chopped

- 1 medium onion, chopped

- 2 tbsp. extra virgin olive oil

- ¼ tsp. sea salt

Directions

Heat extra virgin olive oil in a pan set over medium heat. Stir in onion and sauté over medium low heat for about 15 minutes or until caramelized.

Stir in kale and sauté for 5 more minutes. Season with salt to serve.

Vinegar & Salt Kale Chips

Yields: 6 Servings

Total Time: 27 Minutes

Prep Time: 15 Minutes

Cook Time: 12 Minutes

Ingredients

- 1 tsp. extra virgin olive oil

- 1 head kale, chopped

- 1 tbsp. apple cider vinegar

- ½ tsp. sea salt

Directions

Place kale in a bowl and drizzle with vinegar and extra virgin olive oil; sprinkle with salt and massage the ingredients with hands.

Spread the kale out onto two paper-lined baking sheets and bake at 375°F for about 12 minutes or until crispy.

Let cool for about 10 minutes before serving.

Roasted Balsamic Beets

Yields: 4 Servings

Total Time: 1 Hour 30 Minutes

Prep Time: 15 Minutes

Cook Time: 1 Hour 15 Minutes

Ingredients

- 2 tbsp. extra virgin olive oil
- 1 tbsp. balsamic vinegar
- 3-4 medium beets
- ½ tsp. sea salt

Directions

Scrub the beets and wash well; cut into 6 wedges and place them in a baking dish.

Drizzle the beets with extra virgin olive oil, vinegar and salt and bake, covered, at 375°F for about 1 hour. Uncover and continue baking for 15 more minutes or until almost tender.

Veggie Snack

Yields: 1 Serving

Total Time: 10 Minutes

Prep Time: 10 Minutes

Cook Time: 0 Minutes

Ingredients

- 1 yellow pepper
- 5 stalks celery
- 5 carrots

Directions

Scrub the carrots and rinse under running water.

Rinse celery and yellow pepper; deseed the pepper and chop the veggies into small sticks.

Combine in a bowl and serve.

Sesame Crackers

Yields: 96 Crackers

Total Time: 32 Minutes

Prep Time: 20 Minutes

Cook Time: 12 Minutes

Ingredients

- 1 cup sesame seeds
- 2 tbsp. grapeseed oil
- 2 large free range eggs, beaten
- 1 ½ tsp. sea salt
- 3 cups almond flour, blanched

Directions

Stir together sesame seeds, almond flour, oil, eggs and salt in a large bowl until well combined.

Divide the dough into two portions.

Place each into two baking sheets lined with parchment papers and cover with parchment paper.

Spread the dough between the papers to cover the entire baking sheet and remove the top paper.

With a pizza cutter or knife, cut the dough into 2-inch squares and bake at 350°F until golden brown, for about 12 minutes.

Cool before serving.

Healthy Spiced Nuts

Yields: 4 Servings

Total Time: 20 Minutes

Prep Time: 10 Minutes

Cook Time: 10 Minutes

Ingredients

- 1 tbsp. extra virgin olive oil
- ¼ cup walnuts
- ¼ cup pecans
- ¼ cup almonds
- ½ tsp. sea salt
- ½ tsp. pepper
- ½ tsp. cumin
- 1 tsp. chili powder

Directions

Put the nuts in a skillet set over medium heat and toast until lightly browned.

In the meantime, prepare the spice mixture; combine black pepper, cumin, chili and salt in a bowl.

Coat the toasted nuts with extra virgin olive oil and sprinkle with the spice mixture to serve.

Roasted Asparagus

Yield: 4 Servings

Total Time: 15 Minutes

Prep Time: 5 Minutes

Cook Time: 10 Minutes

Ingredients

- 1 tbsp. extra virgin olive oil
- 1 pound fresh asparagus
- 1 medium lemon, zested
- 1/2 tsp. freshly grated nutmeg
- 1/2 tsp. kosher salt
- ½ tsp. black pepper

Directions

Preheat your oven to 500°F. Arrange asparagus on an aluminum foil and drizzle with extra virgin olive oil; toss until well coated. Spread the asparagus in a single layer and fold the edges of foil to make a tray. Roast the asparagus in the oven for about 5 minutes; toss and continue roasting for 5 minutes more or until browned. Sprinkle the roasted asparagus with nutmeg, salt, zest and pepper to serve.

Sesame Carrots

Yield: 2 Servings

Total Time: 5 Minutes

Prep Time: 5 Minutes

Cook time: N/A

Ingredients

- 1 tbsp. toasted sesame seeds

- 2 cups baby carrots

- Pinch of kosher salt

- Pinch of dried thyme

Directions

In a small bowl, toss the carrots with sesame seeds, salt and thyme.

White bean puree

Yield: 1 Cup

Total Time: 5 Minutes

Prep Time: 5 Minutes

Cook time: N/A

Ingredients

- 1/4 cup garlic-infused olive oil
- 400g can drained cannellini beans, rinsed
- 1 tbsp. lemon juice
- 1/4 cup almond meal

Directions

In a blender, blend lemon juice, almonds, beans and oil until very smooth. Season with pepper and salt to serve.

Raspberry and Apple Crumble

Yield: 4 Servings

Total Time: 1 Hour 15 Minutes

Prep Time: 15 Minutes

Cook time: 1 Hour

Ingredients

- 2 cups rolled oats
- 2 cups apple juice
- 1 cup raspberries
- 5 finely sliced large cooking apples
- 1/2 tsp. cloves
- 2 tsp. cinnamon
- 2 tbsp. honey
- 2 tbsp. butter

Directions

Preheat your oven to 350°F.

Butter a baking dish; arrange raspberries and apple slices in the baking dish and pour over the apple juice.

In a bowl, combine together honey, rolled oats and spices. Using your fingers, cut in the butter to disperse it evenly.

Cover the raspberries and apples with the crumble topping and bake in the preheated oven for about 1 hour. Serve hot.

Buckwheat Crepes with Prune Compote

Yield: 8 Crepes

Total Time: 25 Minutes

Prep Time: 10 Minutes

Cook time: 15 Minutes

Ingredients

- 1/3 cup quinoa flour

- 2/3 cup buckwheat flour

- 1 1/4 cup rice milk

- 2 eggs

- 8 oz. pitted organic dried plums, softened in warm water

- 1 tbsp. apple juice

- 1 tbsp. honey

- Cooking spray, for frying

- 1 tbsp. canola oil

- 1/2 tsp. salt

- 1 cup water

Directions

Whisk the eggs in a bowl. Add canola oil, quinoa flour, buckwheat flour, rice milk, and salt; whisk until well blended.

Set a large skillet over medium heat and spray it with cooking spray.

Pour a third cup of the batter in the skillet and rotate the skillet to evenly coat the bottom with batter. Cook on medium high heat until bubbles appear, for about 2 minutes. Flip the crepe over and cook the other side for 1 minute. Transfer the crepe to a plate and repeat with the remaining batter.

Prepare prune compote: Combine apple juice, sugar, water and prunes in a saucepan set over medium high heat. Bring the mixture to a boil, then reduce heat to medium-low and simmer until the prunes are tender, for about 15 minutes. Remove the compote from heat and let cool a bit, then serve over crepes.

Lettuce Wraps

Yield: 4 Servings

Total Time: 10 Minutes

Prep Time: 10 Minutes

Cook time: N/A

Ingredients

- 8 Romaine lettuce leaves
- 2 tsp. lime juice
- 3 tomatoes, diced
- 2 avocados
- ¼ cup chopped cilantro
- 3 garlic cloves, minced
- ¼ yellow onion, diced
- ½ jalapeno pepper, diced

Directions

Mash avocado in a bowl. Stir in the remaining ingredients until well combined. Spread about 3 tablespoons of the avocado mixture into lettuce leaves and fold to wrap.

Sautéed Shrimp

Yield: 4 Servings

Total Time: 25 Minutes

Prep Time: 10 Minutes

Cook time: 15 Minutes

Ingredients

- ½ pound deveined and peeled shrimp
- 2 tbsp. olive oil
- 1 tbsp. garlic powder
- 2 tbsp. chili powder
- 1 tsp. ground black pepper
- ¼ tsp. cayenne pepper
- ½ tbsp. fresh parsley

Directions

Add extra virgin olive oil to a pan set over medium heat. Stir in shrimp and cook for about 1 minute.

Stir in cayenne pepper, parsley, garlic powder, and chili powder; sauté until shrimp are fully cooked and pink, for about 5 minutes.

Coconut Bread

Yield: 1 Loaf

Total Time: 50 Minutes

Prep Time: 10 Minutes

Cook time: 40 Minutes

Ingredients

- ¾ cup coconut flour, sifted
- 2 tbsp. raw honey
- ½ cup coconut oil
- 6 large eggs
- 1 tsp. baking powder
- ½ tsp. sea salt

Directions

Preheat your oven to 350° F.

Beat together the eggs, salt, honey and oil until well combined. Set aside.

Combine flour and baking powder in a bowl and whisk into the egg mixture until well blended.

Transfer the batter to a loaf pan and bake for about 40 minutes.

Remove the bread from the pan and let cool on a wire rack.

Almond Muffins

Yield: 4 Servings

Total Time: 25 Minutes

Prep Time: 10 Minutes

Cook time: 15 Minutes

Ingredients

- 3 large eggs
- 2 cup coconut, shredded
- 1 cup coconut milk
- 1 cup almonds
- 1 cup almond butter
- 2 tbsp. coconut sap
- ¼ tsp. vanilla

Directions

Preheat your oven to 400° F.

Prepare a muffin tin by lining it with paper liners.

In a bowl, combine all the ingredients and transfer to a muffin tin.

Bake in the preheated oven for about 15 minutes.

Healthy Homemade Applesauce

Yield: 1 Cup

Total Time: 6 Hours 10 Minutes

Prep Time: 10 Minutes

Cook time: 6 Hours

Ingredients

- 3 pounds peeled apples, cored, sliced
- 1 medium lemon, juiced
- ¼ tsp. ground ginger
- ¼ tsp. ground cardamom
- 1 tsp. cinnamon

Directions

Combine all the ingredients in a slow cooker and cook, covered, on low for about 6 hours or until apples are tender.

Transfer the cooked apples to a food processor and pulse until very smooth. Serve chilled or warm.

Tasty Whole Food Bread

Yield: 4 Servings

Total Time: 50 Minutes

Prep Time: 10 Minutes

Cook time: 40 Minutes

Ingredients

- 6 tbsp. ground flax seeds
- 3 tbsp. coconut flour
- 3 cups almond flour
- 11/2 tbsp. apple cider vinegar
- 11/2 tbsp. raw honey
- 11/2 tbsp. melted coconut oil
- 7 large eggs
- 11/2 tsp. baking soda
- ½ tsp. sea salt

Directions

Preheat your oven to 350° F.

Combine flax, flours, sea salt and baking soda in a food processor; mix until well blended. Add in the eggs and continue processing until mixed. Add vinegar, honey and coconut oil and process until well blended.

Coat a bread pan with a generous amount of coconut oil and add the batter.

Bake in the oven until a tester inserted in the center comes out clean, for about 40 minutes.

Cool the bread completely before removing from the pan.

Whole Food Refreshing Drinks

Blueberry Sunflower Smoothie

Ingredients

- 1 tbsp. sunflower seeds
- 1 tbsp. crushed almonds
- ½ lemon
- ½ cup fresh blueberries
- 1 tbsp. honey
- 1 tbsp. chopped mint leaves

Directions

Combine together all the ingredients in a blender. Blend on high speed for 20 seconds or until very smooth. Serve in a glass garnished with more blueberries, lemon slice and a fresh mint leaf.

Catechin-Rich Ice Tea

Yield: 2 Servings

Ingredients

- 2 1/2 tsp. loose green tea leaves

- 2 cups water

- 3 tbsp. freshly squeezed lemon juice

Directions

Boil water in a saucepan.

Place the green tea leaves into a teapot and add the boiled water. Steep for at least 5 minutes and strain the tea. Stir in lemon juice and chill before serving.

Grapefruit Cranberry Sparkler

Ingredients

- 1 cup grapefruit juice

- 1 cup cranberry juice

- Juice of 1/2 lime

- 1 cup sparkling mineral water

Directions

Combine the ingredients in a glass bowl or jar; stir to mix well and divide between two serving glasses. Add ice and garnish each with a slice of lime.

Hot Cocoa

Ingredients

- 1 1/2 tbsp. coconut oil
- ½ tbsp. raw honey
- ½ cup coconut milk
- ½ cup almond milk
- 1 tsp. vanilla
- 1 tbsp. cacao powder, to taste

Directions

Bring coconut milk and almond milk to a gentle boil. Stir in cacao and honey until well blended. Remove the mixture from heat and transfer to a food processor. Add vanilla extract and coconut oil and process until well blended.

Mulled Cider

Ingredients

- 1 lemon, sliced
- 1 orange, sliced
- 1/4 tsp. powdered ginger
- 2 quarts apple cider or juice
- 1/4 tsp. nutmeg
- 6 whole cloves
- 4 sticks cinnamon
- 2 tbsp. raw honey

Directions

Combine all ingredients in a saucepan; bring to a gentle boil. Lower heat and simmer for about 40 minutes. Strain and serve immediately.

Apple Lemonade

Ingredients

- 4 tbsp. lemon juice

- 2 cups apple juice

Directions

Combine the ingredients and chill before serving. Serve over ice.

Strawberry Lemonade

Ingredients

- 2 lemons sliced

- 1 cup lemon juice

- 1 tbsp. honey

- 1 cup strawberries

- 1 cup strawberries

- 8 cups water

Directions

Soak the strawberries in a container with 4 cups of water for at least 3 hours.

Combine sliced lemons, lemon juice and water in a container and chill for at least 3 hours. Mix the two containers together and stir in honey. Serve chilled.

Lime Coconut Fizz Cooler

Ingredients

- 1 cup sparkling water

- 2 tbsp. raw honey

- ½ cup thick coconut milk

- ½ cup lime juice

- 1 cup ice

For garnishes

- More sliced limes

- Fresh mint

Directions

Blend together honey, coconut milk, lime juice and ice cubes in a blender until very smooth. Stir on sparkling water

Serve the coconut lime fizz into the glasses and serve immediately garnished with mint and limes.

Basil, Ginger and Lemon Iced Tea

Ingredients

- 9 cups boiling water

- 3 tbsp. honey

- 3/4 cup basil leaves

- 5 ginger coins

- ½ cup lemon juice

Directions

Combine lemon juice, basil and ginger coins in a pitcher. Add boiling water and stir until well combined. Stir in honey and let sit until cool. Remove basil and ginger and serve with ice.

Cacao Smoothie w/ Macadamias

Ingredients

- 1 tbsp. ground chia seeds
- 2 tbsp. raw cacao powder
- 6-8 macadamia nuts
- 1 cup almond milk
- 3 or 4 dates, pitted
- 1/2 cup baby spinach
- 1 ripe banana

Directions

Blend together all the ingredients in a blender until very smooth.

Serving in a glass sprinkled with cacao powder.

Raspberry Lemonade

Ingredients

- 3/4 cup honey

- 1/2 cup lemon juice

- 1 pint raspberries

- 8 cups water

- 1 cup ice

Directions

Combine honey, lemon juice, raspberries and 1 cup of water in a pan set over medium heat; bring the mixture to a gentle boil, stirring to dissolve honey.

Strain the mixture into a serving glass and stir in the remaining water and ice.

Serve cold.

Creamy Peach Smoothie

Ingredients

- 1 cup Coconut milk

- 2 peaches

- Pinch of cinnamon

- 1 cup Ice

- Dash of vanilla extract

Directions

Blend together all the ingredients until very smooth. Serve immediately.

Spice Tea

Ingredients

- 1 cup hot water

- ½ tsp. coriander

- ½ tsp. fennel

- ½ tsp. cumin

Directions

Combine the ingredients and let sit for about 5 minutes. Strain and drink immediately.

Hydration Juice

Ingredients

- 1/4 organic beet

- 2 organic apples

- 2-3 large cucumbers

- Organic mint

Directions

In a juicer, juice everything together; stir in ice and serve garnished with mint sprigs.

Matcha Pineapple Mango Smoothie

Ingredients

- 1/2 to 1 cup water
- 1 cup pineapple
- 1 tbsp. pineapple juice
- 1 cup frozen mango chunks
- 1 tsp. honey
- 1 tbsp. protein powder
- 1.25 tsp. matcha green tea

Directions

Chop up all the fresh fruit and blend all together in a blender. Enjoy!

Body Cleaner

Total Time: 5 minutes

Yield: 2 Servings

Ingredients:

- 1 knob ginger

- 1/2 lemon

- 1 medium beet

- 1 cup fresh cilantro

- 6 celery stalks

Directions:

Juice all the ingredients through a vegetable juicer and stir to mix well. Enjoy!

Liver Detox Juice

Ingredients:

- 1 organic beet, peeled
- ½ organic lemon, peeled
- ½ inch ginger root
- 2 organic red apples, chopped
- 3 organic carrots, peeled
- 6 organic kale leaves

Directions:

Place all the ingredients in a juicer and juice. Stir to mix well and serve with ice cubes.

Parting Shot...

I would like to express my gratitude once more for purchasing this whole diet book.

I hope it helps you understand the principles of healthy living, what you should do to restore balance in your entire being and the fact that all you need to be healed and feel whole again is fresh, healthy, natural and wholesome food. Not food that's been sitting on a shelf in a box for over 2 months and that's still going to be safe for consumption for the next six months!

The next step is to focus on getting the right attitude and frame of mind to help you make the necessary eating and lifestyle changes that will stick with you from now henceforth.

You may not have tried this diet before, but what's there to lose if not lots to gain? All the best in your 30 day whole food diet challenge!

161

www.ingramcontent.com/pod-product-compliance
Lightning Source LLC
Chambersburg PA
CBHW071329310526
45789CB00017B/2013